Special Delivery

SPECIAL DELIVERY

The Choices Are Yours

Rahima Baldwin Dancy

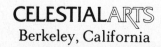
CELESTIALARTS
Berkeley, California

Celestial Arts
P.O. Box 7327
Berkeley, California 94707

Cover design: Ken Scott

Cover photograph: Harriette Hartigan/Artemis

Illustrations: Abigail Dunn
Photographs: Wahhab Baldwin 1978; except pages
50, 51, Figures 4-5 through 4-10, Billy Schaffner;
page 56, Figure 5-1; page 61, Figure 5-9; and page 144,
Figure 10-3, James Radkins

First Printing, February 1979
Revised, October 1986
Made in the United States of America

Library of Congress Cataloging in Publication Data

Baldwin, Rahima, 1949-
  Special delivery.

  Bibliography: p.
  Includes index.
  1. Natural childbirth   2. Childbirth at home.
I. Title
RG661.B34   618.4'5   78-61611
ISBN 0-89087-934-6

    16 17 — 00

ACKNOWLEDGEMENTS

When I began to investigate birth in 1971, the first author I encountered was Sheila Kitzinger. I still remember writing her a long letter expressing my relief that birth didn't have to be a gruelling ordeal or a medical nightmare. When I learned that I was living only a few miles from her in the English countryside, I arranged to attend her classes with the National Childbirth Trust. Her themes of the psychology and sensuality of birth and the possibility of homebirth became my own.

Over the intervening years, I feel privileged to have met others in the field of birth and to have shared our common ideals—Dr. Frederick LeBoyer, Tonya Brooks, Gayle Peterson and Lewis Mehl, Nancy Cohen and Claudia Panuthos.

I would also like to thank the couples in Colorado who were giving birth at home in the 1970s (some of whose accounts you will read in this book), and who invited those of us studying birth to be present and to become midwives in the process. Margaret Fiedler and her friends and family, who were exploring birth in Mexico, also had a profound effect on my attitudes toward birth, life and children. Margaret was always there reminding us that birth is a part of life, not a series of separate emergencies.

Special Delivery grew out of a manual I had written for classes and to accompany the tape series for couples who lived too far away to attend. The final book was written in the hills of Guerrero, Mexico at the home of Dr. Mickey Rostaker and Cathy Ellis, a Canadian midwife. I am still grateful for all the books and articles on birthing that had been brought together there by Mickey. And I want to thank Wahhab for writing the book with me during those crazy six weeks when we pecked away at two manual typewriters every day from 9 in the morning until 11 at night while our two small children somehow amused themselves. Thanks also go to Dr. Julie Carpenter, of Boulder, Colorado for reading the text for medical accuracy.

And, finally, I would like to thank David Hinds of Celestial Arts for his integrity and support in keeping *Special Delivery* alive and available.

PREFACE to the FIRST EDITION

As a childbirth educator, I have observed in recent years a major shift in what women and couples are seeking in their births. An increasing number of couples no longer accept birth as a medical procedure which must be supervised by an expert whose word is to be acted upon without question. Instead, they see birth as a natural process, for which, no matter how much technical help they accept, they themselves remain ultimately responsible.

Any birth carried out with this awareness, with the focus on the people rather than on the technology, on the process rather than on the goal, is a special delivery. This is true whether the setting is the parents' home, a hospital or a birth center.

This book has been written to encourage parents to be steadfast in what they already feel—that they should understand birth, make it an integral part of their lives, a joyous process throughout which they can maintain a sense of dignity and self-determinism. It is based on the conviction that since parents are going to make choices for themselves in any event, they should be given the fullest information and tools possible for the task they are undertaking: giving birth with the greatest safety and emotional and spiritual fulfillment for the baby, mother, and everyone present.

The major focus of the book is on homebirth, growing out of my work with hundreds of couples as president of Informed Homebirth, a national organization dedicated to furthering safe alternatives in childbirth. But wherever you choose to give birth, whether home, birth center or hospital, if you recognize that no one but you can be responsible for the experience you are going to have, you will benefit by the practical information in *Special Delivery*.

This is a practical book, including many pages in workbook format, self-quizzes and other aids for helping you to understand all aspects of birth. I have also written it as a dialogue, since I do not wish to depersonalize our relationships. And although it is addressed to the mother-to-be, it is certainly a useful tool for fathers-to-be, birth attendants, doctors, and everyone concerned with the quality of birth.

After struggling with the unfortunate organization of pronouns in the English language, I finally decided to use feminine pronouns for birth attendants and masculine and feminine pronouns for babies, on some pages referring to the baby as "he" and on others as "she." And I have used the words "partner," "husband" and "father" interchangeably, while still recognizing that there are a great variety of living arrangements. Although this book is oriented toward couples, I know that an increasing number of women are deciding to give birth without being together with a man. Whatever your particular situation, this book can help prepare you for a responsible and joyous birth experience surrounded by people you love.

I hope this book will make it easier for you to get the information you need and will encourage you to continually examine your own ideas and ideals. I'd be glad to hear from you with questions or comments about this book, about our classes, tape series, teacher training program or other services. A convenient questionnaire is included at the end of the book if you would like further information. Best wishes for your birth!

Rahima Baldwin
July, 1978
Boulder, Colorado

PREFACE to the SECOND EDITION

In the years since *Special Delivery* was first published, there have been many changes in birth in this country. Birth centers have flourished and thus have contributed to the adoption of more family-centered practices in standard hospital birth. The practice of midwifery has spread, as more and more states allow empirical as well as nurse midwives to attend births. And the homebirth movement has grown and matured, making this option more available and contributing what it has learned about normal birth to the practices of both birth centers and hospitals.

In a similar way, Informed Homebirth has grown from a local attempt to meet the need for information on alternatives in birth to a national organization that has trained over 1000 childbirth educators and helped countless couples since it was founded in 1977. Along the way it added the second name, Informed Birth and Parenting, to take the message of parent responsibility, nonintervention, reclaiming second stage, and so forth, to all women regardless of where they choose to give birth.

This revision of *Special Delivery* reflects that same change, a desire to make what we in homebirth have learned about women and birth more accessible to all women. It therefore includes added sections on hospital options to help women get what they want within the system as well as outside of it. But women who will be birthing in a conventional hospital are also referred to additional resources, because some environments require more watchfulness than others to assure what you want.

Revising a book is an exercise in determining what is temporal and what is abiding. Most of the book remains unchanged, but material has been updated as needed and we have included new developments such as cesarean prevention and working with the emotional aspects of birth, although both these topics are covered in far greater detail in *Pregnant Feelings* (written together with Terra Palmarini). It can be seen as a companion volume to *Special Delivery*, for it explores the psychological aspects of birthing, just as this book covers its practical aspects.

It is an exciting time to be having a baby, because so many more options and choices are available than ever before. That trend will accelerate as women continue to take back birth, both as mothers and as attendants. We need to be informed, to recognize our vulnerability and our strengths, and to know that it is possible to have the kind of birth we want for ourselves and our babies. This book is designed to give you the information and the awareness you need to make your own best choices.

Rahima Baldwin
October 1986
Ann Arbor, Michigan

Contents

Special Delivery

CHAPTER ONE

The New Consciousness in Birth

THE HOMEBIRTH REVOLUTION

Despite the fact that almost all of the people now alive in the world were born at home,[1] the homebirth movement in the United States, which I call the new homebirth, is completely revolutionary, something which has never before happened in human history. We now find that women, together with their partners, are giving birth at home as safely and with fewer complications than in the average hospital birth,[2] and are finding it a joyous process, indeed a peak experience in their lives.

This joyful experience of birth is the keynote of the new homebirth. Indeed the current return to home deliveries is not a return at all, because it involves a new *consciousness* of birth. When your great-grandmother gave birth at home, she may have done so stoically or moaning and praying that it would soon be over. She believed that the pains of childbirth were women's lot and was embarrassed before her husband, who either paced nervously downstairs, or went out to get drunk. After participating in just such births in rural Mexico, I am strengthened in the conviction that there is no such thing as "natural childbirth"—a woman either follows her cultural conditioning or makes the leap to a new realization which, although still only recognized by a minority of women, is now available to us all.

The new homebirth is a completely new response to birth, a recognition that what we need to vitalize our lives, save our humanity, and renew our sensitivity, is to choose actively to *feel* and to know ourselves, our lives, our births, our deaths. Through this realization, women are not only actively giving birth with dignity and joy, but are also reclaiming their birthright—the right to be self-determined and recognized, especially in the uniquely feminine act of giving birth.

The second key to the new homebirth is women's desire to assume active responsibility for their bodies, their lives and their birth experiences. Instead of showing a blind dependency on experts, passively allowing doctors to impose their authority on them, couples are informing themselves as much as possible and selecting birth attendants who will help *them* in their actions—attendants who are not only medically skilled, but also sensitive and aware of the emotional and psychological qualities of birth. For people are coming to know in their hearts that the *way* in which something is done may be even more important than *what* is done, and they have found that the medical establishment has placed a very low priority on the emotional and spiritual experiences of the people it serves. This has forced couples to find new types of birth attendants, to learn for themselves what has formerly been the sacred domain of the experts, and to come to trust the knowledge of their own bodies, minds and intuitions.

The third key, then, in understanding the new homebirth is the recognition that birth is a spiritual process, one which has lasting psychological and physiological effects. Parents are demanding, from the moment of birth, the recognition that their child is a whole and sensitive person to be treated with care and respect. And although these realizations have so far been consciously formulated only by a minority of parents, the

---

[1]Marion Sousa claims, "Fully 98 percent of the people now alive were born at home." *Childbirth at Home* (New York: Bantam, 1977), p. 15.

[2]See pp. 4–7 for documentation.

force of this realization has been so strong that it has already affected changes in many hospitals' procedures and will continue to transform the American way of birth.

RECLAIMING BIRTH:
HISTORICAL ROOTS OF THE CHANGE

The reclaiming of the birth experience by women has been fueled by prepared childbirth classes and ignited by books such as Suzanne Arms' *Immaculate Deception*.[3] It has transformed hospitals, led to the establishment of birth centers, and been the driving force behind the new homebirth. The recognition is emerging everywhere: birth is a joyful and spiritual process with lasting impact on everyone involved. To see how radical this statement really is, we have only to glance at the history of birth in the West.

For centuries birth was not only a painful, but also a dangerous prospect. The invention of forceps in 1598 began the gradual shift towards safer births, but also resulted in births being turned over to specialists, men who guarded the secret of forceps not only from women but from discovery by other doctors.

Queen Victoria's radical choice of using chloroform at the birth of Prince Leopold in 1853 was the start of overcoming the conviction, here expressed by a minister in 1855, that

> Pain during childbirth is, in the majority of cases, even desirable!. . .Yet there are those bold enough to administer the vapor of ether, even at this critical juncture, forgetting it has been ordered that "in sorrow shall she bring forth."[4]

But the introduction of anesthetics didn't really change the conviction that birth was painful, and it left women even more passive and completely dependent on their obstetrician to deliver their baby.

The discovery by Semmelweis in the mid-nineteenth century that lack of antiseptic technique was responsible for the tremendous death rate in hospitals from "childbed fever" helped to make hospital births safer than they had been (although American hospitals were especially slow in adopting sterile methods, not using them for more than three decades after Semmelweis' discoveries).

By the 1930s, an increasing number of births were being done in hospitals and more and more drugs were being used. In 1935, 37 percent of U.S. births were in hospitals. By 1950 the percentage had risen to 88 percent, and by 1960 it had reached 96 percent.[5] Doctors discouraged homebirths because technicalization of birth and the shortage of civilian doctors during World War II required the equipment and centralization of the hospital environment. Birth had become a technological process, requiring experts to bring the baby out of a mother who was unconscious on the delivery table.

The counterswing to this trend has its roots in Grantly Dick-Read's *Childbirth Without Fear*, published in 1933 in England and in 1945 in America. But it was Marjorie Carmel's *Thank You, Dr. Lamaze* (1956) which first brought a large number of Americans the message that a woman could approach childbirth consciously and with dignity, without depending on drugs.

This was a remarkable shift, allowing women to make such statements as, "I gave birth to Thomas by the psychoprophylactic method called childbirth without pain. When friends say to me, 'Well, did you feel nothing?' I reply, 'Quite the opposite, I felt everything, and that is the wonderful part of it . . . the amazing experience in which each second has remained imprinted on my memory and in which pain has simply found no place.' "[6]

The next major step forward we owe to Dr. Robert Bradley, whose *Husband-Coached Childbirth* made the father an integral part of the birthing team and allowed him not only to be present but also to take an active role in the birth of his child.

But even though prepared childbirth leaves the woman awake and aware, it does so within a framework in which she is still a patient, under the authority of a doctor and subject to the schedules and indignities of hospital routine. The woman has not yet truly been recognized as the central, and hence responsible, person in the act of birth. Lamaze classes in this country, despite all the good they have done, have often become so watered down that neither obstetricians nor women feel that spinal anesthesia is incompatible with prepared childbirth. Although most Lamaze teachers will discuss how to ward off unwanted anesthesia, many ask for a permission slip from the woman's doctor to attend classes, then urge her not to be a martyr and to accept anesthesia if it hurts, rather than dealing squarely with the issues of feeling and experiencing her baby being born, and the effects of anesthesia on the baby.

[3] For complete information on all books mentioned herein, see the bibliography at the end of the book.

[4] Quoted in Theodore Cianfrani, *A Short History of Obstetrics and Gynecology* (Springfield, Ill: Charles Thomas, 1960), p. 293.

[5] Neal Devitt, "The Transition from Home to Hospital Birth in the United States, 1930–1960," *Birth and the Family Journal* 4 (Summer 1977): 47.

[6] Fernand Lamaze, *Painless Childbirth: The Lamaze Method* (New York: Pocket Books, 1972), p. 17.

This compromise with anesthetics (unless necessitated by a *medical* emergency) is a far cry from Dr. Lamaze's injunction:

> Those who still maintain that anesthesia should be used during delivery can never have seen the face of a woman who has herself brought her child into the world. No obstetrician or midwife can forget that face, radiant with joy and full of pride, as the mother sees her child being born.[7]

I will add, sees and feels her baby being born *by her own efforts*, not by forceps, which are usually necessary with regional anesthesia.

And while students of the Bradley Method, on the other hand, do succeed in giving birth without drugs in over 90 percent of cases, Dr. Bradley still regards the "little woman" as a little girl who is "nuttier than a fruitcake" during pregnancy[8] and needs to follow her husband's and obstetrician's more rational leads in areas such as routine episiotomy, for example.

NATURE OF THE CHANGE

Thus we see that self-awareness is not yet intrinsically present in prepared childbirth classes in this country. The completely new realization is the recognition by the couple that they themselves are the pivot and focus, the responsible parties and the intentional agents, of the birth process. As such they are seeking help, both inside and outside the medical system, in trying to understand themselves and birth, and they deserve all the respect, knowledge and acknowledgment that can be given them by friends, childbirth educators and birth attendants.

Does this mean they have turned their backs on medicine, technology and medical expertise? No, not at all. Couples involved with homebirth today are seeking to be informed, to make responsible decisions, and to have a skilled birth attendant present who is willing to work with them. They are seeking and demanding quality prenatal care, and if doctors are refusing them because of their plans to have a home delivery, they are forming their own self-help prenatal clinics or starting birth centers. People are coming to trust their bodies and their own ability to learn and make informed decisions. They are coming to feel that medical technology should be reserved for those cases in which it is required (i.e., high-risk pregnancies, which can be detected through prenatal care, and unforeseen complications, which occur in five to ten percent of prepared homebirths).

However, as is the case with all revolutions in consciousness, the people are changing faster than the institutions, and there are more couples involved with the new homebirth than there are medical people prepared to help them. Couples are searching for skilled birth attendants who not only regard birth as a normal physiological process, but who also encourage couples to share in decision-making rather than being "patients." Since so few doctors are either trained in normal birth[9] or willing to enter into this new relationship with women, couples are turning to midwives as the "guardians of normal birth" and asking that doctors fulfill their role of medical experts by providing backup in the small percentage of births requiring medical intervention.

Although they are not turning their backs on technology, parents involved with the new homebirth have realized what doctors in Holland have always known: that birth is a natural human function, which in general works best if not meddled with (see Kloosterman's discussion, p. 5). Recently the evidence has been multiplying that the technological approach to birth not only robs a woman of a unique experience, but that it also has many health disadvantages. Just as people are coming to know that a blind devotion to industrial technology which does not recognize the integrity of the earth may become lethal, so we are coming to know that an overly medical approach to health has *iatrogenic*, or self-induced, counter-productive results.[10] The new homebirth is an ecology of the body and an expansion of the spirit.

In summary, the driving force behind the new homebirth is the realization that, in order to be fully alive, it is necessary for us to participate actively in what we do, to bring our consciousness, feelings, sense of responsibility and decision-making ability to bear as fully as possible in every action of our daily lives, and especially in an event as momentous as birth.

THE ADVANTAGES OF HOMEBIRTH

You don't have to have your baby at home to participate in this new consciousness. Some women or couples may choose to deliver in a birth center or hospital, either because of risk factors or because they feel more comfortable in an environment where many factors are predetermined and emergency equipment is close at

---

[7]*Ibid.*, p. 173.

[8]Robert Bradley, *Husband-Coached Childbirth* (New York: Harper & Row, 1974), p. 117.

[9]Many doctors who have become involved with homebirth have attended homebirths with midwives and learned from them the confidence and techniques of normal birth, which are sadly lacking in the curricula of medical schools and missing from the wards of teaching hospitals.

[10]For a discussion of iatrogenesis, see Ivan Illich's *Medical Nemesis: The Expropriation of Health* (New York: Pantheon, 1976).

hand. Wherever you give birth, I urge you to explore what it means to take responsibility and to be an informed medical "consumer" (or, better yet, "determiner").

I certainly do not advocate homebirth for everyone. Rather, I recommend that you give birth in the place where you feel best. But to help balance the scales against the counter-arguments that are so common, I would like to enumerate some of the advantages of giving birth at home.

SELF-DETERMINISM

In the comfort of your own home, you are not reduced to the status of a patient. You are in charge. You can do what you want in the way you want. Everyone is present at your request, including birth attendants, who are more likely to view birth as a normal process and share knowledge and decision-making with you.

STRENGTHENING OF THE FAMILY

The father can take an active role in the birth, rather than being "allowed" to be present in the delivery room. You can share in the intimacy of labor and birth without being interrupted by changing shifts of nurses or interns coming in to do exams. Some midwives will even help the father catch the baby as the mother delivers her to the outside world. If you choose, your other children can share in the birth and immediately bond with the baby, and no one has to be separated after the birth. The birth is an integrated part of your lives.

NO UNNECESSARY MEDICAL INTERVENTION

You can avoid the dangers and discomfort of routine spinal anesthesia and accompanying forceps, routine electronic fetal monitoring, use of pitocin or relaxants, and routine episiotomy. You do not require a pubic shave, routine enema or IV drip. You don't need to interrupt your rhythms by going from home to hospital or from labor bed to delivery room. You and your labor are granted much more individuality at home. In short, your baby is born without medical procedures which can be valuable in high-risk cases but which, when used on the normal mother and baby, can actually jeopardize the health of both.

CHOICE OF POSITION FOR LABOR AND BIRTH

Delivering on a narrow table with your legs strapped into stirrups (in the hospital in Los Angeles where I taught Lamaze classes they still strapped your wrists down as well) is not only uncomfortable and degrading but is also the worst position for your perineal muscles and almost necessitates an episiotomy (cutting of the birth canal) to avoid tearing. Delivering in a more relaxed position at home with a skilled birth attendant, you almost never need an episiotomy (standard in 95 percent of hospital births) and you rarely tear. You can also be on your hands and knees or relax in the bathtub during labor if they help you feel comfortable, and squatting can often overcome lack of progress without the need for drugs or forceps.

ADVANTAGES FOR BABY

The baby is born without being drugged and dragged out by forceps. He or she is welcomed into a loving environment where the trauma of birth is eased by soft lights, gentle touch and reassurance. Immediately after the birth your baby can nurse and can bond with you both instead of being whisked off to be bathed, weighed, banded, footprinted, and so forth. Your baby is treated as an individual, and his or her uniqueness is clearly recognized and honored.

There is less chance of infection at home than in a hospital nursery, and your baby's every need is instantly satisfied when she or he is with you rather than being one of many under a nurse's care. Breastfeeding on demand helps your milk come in and prevents some common problems of nursing. It also results in a happier and more secure baby who doesn't experience separation, or having to wait for what must seem like eternity when she or he is hungry or in pain or lonely.

FOCUS ON QUALITY

You have the total attention of your birth attendant, rather than thirty minutes of your obstetrician's time and occasional help from nurses. Because your birth is the only thing happening in your home, the total focus of attention and energy of everyone present can be directed towards creating the emotional qualities you want. You are surrounded and assisted by people who love you, not by strangers. If you are more comfortable and more relaxed at home, your labor will go better.

The emotional, spiritual and transforming qualities are not something we have to add to birth—they are inherent in the nature and magnitude of this holy event. If we open to these qualities, we cannot help being transformed.

BUT IS HOMEBIRTH SAFE?

A common misconception, fostered by well-meaning medical professionals, is that homebirth poses grave risks and dangers, while hospitals, with their immense arsenal of equipment and emergency procedures, provide the safest birth money can buy. So strongly do they feel this that several state medical associations have been contemplating revoking licenses of physicians who participate in out-of-hospital births, and some hospitals revoke hospital privileges to any on their staff who even offer assistance to homebirth couples.

However, as the homebirth movement matures and more studies are completed on maternal and infant outcome, the results demonstrate that prepared homebirths (with prenatal care and a skilled birth attendant) not only have a mortality rate as good as or better than hospital births, but have a much *better* record in terms of complications and damage to the baby.

How can this be true? How can it be that all the tools of modern medicine don't improve on the simplicity of a homebirth?

Every farmer and veterinarian knows that interfering with an animal in labor will cause problems in the birth, but our medical system does not apply the wisdom of this benign non-interference to humans. Rather, it is moving towards ever-greater use of dangerous medical and surgical procedures (which may be helpful in high-risk situations) on what should be normal mothers and babies.

For example, the cesarean rate in U.S. hospitals ranges from 10 percent to nearly 50 percent, while the rate at The Farm in Tennessee, where prenatal care and delivery are done at home by "empirical" midwives, is only 1.5 percent. And in considering other populations as a whole, we find the cesarean ratio to be between two and five percent in Holland and England. There is abundant evidence of the damage and dangers inherent in cesarean sections, including risks of anesthesia, higher risk of pelvic infection, and risk of complications for the baby.[11] But rather than working to reduce the cesarean rate, the medical profession is encouraging c-sections by adopting routine use of electronic fetal monitoring.

The electronic fetal monitor (EFM) is perhaps the outstanding current example of needless and harmful meddling in normal labor. It restricts the mother's movement and an internal monitor often involves premature artificial rupture of the amniotic sac and insertion of an electrode puncturing the baby's scalp. Studies such as that of Haverkamp[12] have shown that the use of

EFM triples the cesarean rate *while not providing a single area of improved outcome.*

The unfortunate dehumanization and mechanization of birth by American hospitals is thoroughly discussed by Doris Haire in *The Cultural Warping of Childbirth* and Suzanne Arms in *Immaculate Deception.* I will cite only one other example, the use of forceps in up to 65 percent of American hospital births. The incredibly high forceps rate in this country is necessitated by the lithotomy position for delivery, the use of regional anesthesia, and by the belief (not shared in other countries) that forceps have no deleterious effect on the baby.

The application of forceps and other procedures is being done with such vigor in an effort to improve maternal and infant outcome, and yet that doesn't happen—as evidenced by the fact that there are sixteen countries which have better infant mortality rates than the United States.[13]

In The Netherlands, which had the third lowest rate of infant mortality in 1973, about two-thirds of all babies were born at home with trained midwives usually doing the deliveries. Transfers to the hospital occurred at a rate of less than 2 percent for multiparas and about 8 percent for primiparas (mothers with first babies). Holland's cesarean rate was only 2.3 percent, and forceps were used only in about 3 percent of the births.[14]

OBSTETRICS IN HOLLAND

Dr. G. J. Kloosterman, as chief of obstetrics and gynecology at Amsterdam University, described the philosophy upon which Dutch obstetrics is so successfully based:

> (1) Childbirth in itself, even in human beings, is a natural phenomenon that in the large majority of all cases needs no interference whatsoever; only close observation, moral support and protection against human meddlesomeness.
>
> (2) A healthy woman who delivers spontaneously performs in the large majority of all cases a job that cannot be improved.
>
> (3) This job can be done in the best way if the woman is self-confident and stays in a surrounding where she is the real center (as for example, in her own home).

[11]A recent study by two Brown University researchers in Rhode Island has shown that the risk of maternal death is twenty-six times greater with a cesarean birth than it is for women who deliver vaginally. This was found in an eleven-year study of maternal death in cesarean sections by Dr. John R. Evrand and Dr. Edwin M. Gold and reported in the Journal of *Obstetrics and Gynecology.* The percentage of cesarean births doubled in Rhode Island between 1965 and 1975, which is similar to the pattern nationally. Reported in *NAPSAC News,* Vol. 3, No. 3, Summer, 1978, p. 19.

[12]Haverkamp's study and other data on EFM from Dr. Frederic Ettner, "Hospital Obstetrics: Do the Benefits Outweigh the Risks?" in

21st Century Obstetrics Now! (Chapel Hill, N.C., NAPSAC, 1977), pp. 147-62. His list of complications induced by EFM includes scalp abcesses and cellulitis, infection, fear and pain in the mother, and fetal distress.

[13]Infant mortality figures for 1982 from Wegman, M.E. *Annual Summary of Vital Statistics,* Pediatrics, 74:6:981-90, December 1984.

[14]"Obstetrics in the Netherlands: A Survival or a Challenge?" address by G. J. Kloosterman, M.D. before the Meiu Tunbridge Wells Meeting, 1975.

(4) It is possible during pregnancy, by thorough prenatal care, to divide the expectant mothers into two groups: a large one that shows no recognizable symptoms of pathology (the so-called low-risk group) and a much smaller one in which there are signs of slight or gross abnormalities.

(5) Only this last group, the group at risk, belongs in a highly qualified hospital under the care of specialists.[15]

Sweden, which often has the lowest infant mortality rate, has almost all births occurring in the hospital, so it obviously is not the location *per se* that is at issue. Rather, it is the attitudes, procedures and approach toward birth that determine outcome and cause problems and dissatisfaction with hospital birth (it must be noted that in Sweden, all normal births use the Lamaze techniques with no anesthesia and are attended by midwives in the hospital). Sweden, Holland, and the other five countries with the lowest infant immortality rates are the developed countries of the world with the largest proportions of midwives.

Until the training and orientation of American doctors undergoes a profound shift in these areas, any attempt to humanize the hospitals by adding flowered wallpaper and an easy chair, while still welcome, will remain only superficial and fail to address the real issues. Hospital procedures can be life-saving when needed, but their routine application to low-risk births can be detrimental to the health of both mother and baby, as well as being emotionally unsatisfying for the mother and other members of the family.

HOMEBIRTH SAFETY IN THE UNITED STATES

As already mentioned, the percentage of U.S. births taking place in hospitals rose from 37 percent to 96 percent between 1935 and 1960. Since outcomes improved considerably during this period as well, doctors often point to this as an indication of the effectiveness of their approach. In fact, however, homebirths were becoming safer during this period as well. A recent analysis of the studies done between 1930 and 1960 shows that even then the incidence of birth injuries and obstetric mortality was greater in hospitals than in homebirths—despite the poverty, ill health and frequent high-risk conditions of the women who delivered at home.[16]

For example, the Chicago Maternity Center delivered more than 12,000 babies at home without a single maternal death (despite the fact that fully 80 percent or more of home deliveries in poverty areas are high-risk births); at the same time the maternal death rate in hospitals was 2 per 1,000.

Despite all the brouhaha raised by the medical profession over techniques of labor and delivery, by far the most important factors in determining birth outcome are nutrition, prenatal care and preparation (like prepared childbirth classes). In fact, 66 percent of our perinatal mortality is due to low birth weight, and although medical science has improved in keeping premature and low birth weight babies alive, Devitt states that 75 percent of the recent reduction in neonatal mortality is due to the reduction in the rate of low birth weight, *not to changes in obstetrical care.*[17]

HOMEBIRTH VS. HOSPITAL BIRTH: THE MEHL STUDY

The largest scientific study comparing outcomes of homebirth with hospital birth is Dr. Lewis Mehl and associates' "Home Birth Versus Hospital Birth: Comparisons of Outcomes of Matched Populations."[18] In the study, 1046 homebirths were compared with 1046 hospital births of equivalent populations in the U.S. For each home-delivered patient, a hospital-delivered patient was matched for age, length of gestation, parity, risk factor score, education and socio-economic status, race, presentation of the baby and individual major risk factors. The homebirth population had trained attendants and prenatal care.

Their study shows a three times greater likelihood of cesarean operation if couples gave birth in a hospital instead of at home with the hospital standing by. The data from their hospital population revealed twenty times more forceps, twice as much use of oxytocin to accelerate or induce labor, greater use of analgesia and anesthesia, and nine times greater incidence of episiotomy (while at the same time having more severe tears in need of major repair). The hospital sample showed six times more infant distress in labor, five times more cases of maternal high blood pressure, and three times greater incidence of postpartum hemorrhage. There was four times more infection among the newborn; three times more babies needed help to begin breathing. While the hospital sample had thirty cases of birth injuries, including skull fractures, facial nerve palsies, brachial nerve injuries and severe cephalohematomas, there were no such injuries at home.

The infant death rate of their study was low in both cases and essentially the same. There were no maternal

[15]*Ibid.*

[16]Neal Devitt, *op.cit.*, pp. 47–58.

[17]Neal Devitt, *op. cit.*, p. 51.

[18]Presented on October 20, 1976 before the 104th annual meeting of the American Public Health Association. For further information, contact the Institute for Childbirth and Family Research, 2522 Dana St., Suite 201, Berkeley, CA 94704.

deaths for either home or hospital. The main differences were in the significant improvement of the mother's and baby's health if the couple planned a homebirth, and this was true despite the fact that the homebirth statistics of their study included those couples who began labor at home but ultimately needed to be transferred to the hospital.

STATISTICS FROM THE FARM, SUMMERTOWN, TENNESSEE

Perhaps the best example of a self-contained system of prepared homebirth within the United States is provided by The Farm, an intentional spiritual community founded and led by Stephen Gaskin. Beginning with his wife, Ina May Gaskin, The Farm gradually evolved a group of self-trained or "empirical" midwives. They published their statistics for the 1000 births managed by The Farm midwives between October 1970 and March 1979. These statistics include seventy-five deliveries the midwives considered high-risk and which delivered in the hospital or maternity center.

Of the 1000 births, 43 percent were babies of first-time mothers (primipara). Of all the births 93 percent were delivered at home by the midwives; there were only fifteen cesarean sections (1.5 percent) and three forceps births (0.3 percent). The largest baby they delivered weighed 11 lbs. 4 oz., and the smallest living baby, 2 lbs. 10½ oz. They have never had a mother die, and their total number of perinatal deaths (babies dying between 28 weeks gestation through 28 days after birth) was fifteen, a rate of 15/1000, which is lower than most hospitals.

Of their thirty-two breech births (buttocks first), seventeen were first-time mothers and only one required a cesarean. The most recent eighteen were all done at home or in The Farm Maternity Center. All but two of the breeches were done without anesthesia, and half were done with no episiotomy. This is in dramatic contrast to the practice in most hospitals which calls for an automatic cesarean for breech births, with anesthesia and forceps for those who do delivery vaginally. Later statistics for 1723 births showed a cesarean rate of 4.2 percent, a forceps rate of .46 percent and perinatal mortality of 10.4/1000.

The Farm attributes some of their outstanding statistics to their vegetarian diet and healthy lifestyle. In birth they focus on the psychological and spiritual aspects and on having strong husband-wife and mother-midwife relationships.[19]

OTHER RECENT STUDIES

An annotated bibliography of twelve medical and scientific publications from 1969 to 1985 that support midwifery and homebirth is available from NAPSAC International, Rt. 1, Box 646, Marble Hill, MO 63764. Several of the articles refute the press release issued by the American Medical Association in 1979 showing a two to five times higher infant mortality rate for out of hospital births in many states.[20] This press release, often erroneously labelled a "study," included unplanned, premature and taxicab births and miscarriages along with planned out-of-hospital births. Studies in North Carolina and Kentucky both show that planned out-of-hospital births have much better outcomes than unplanned ones and outcomes comparable to the hospital population.[21]

WHAT ABOUT YOU?

We have just discussed birth statistics at some length. But when you have your baby, you are not a statistic. No one can say with absolute certainty that because most cases like yours have gone well, yours will; or, conversely, that just because your case is "high-risk" it will have problems. Since there are no guarantees in birth, your individual situation will be governed by your actions and decisions during pregnancy and at the time of birth and by forces coming together in that particular moment, not by national averages.

It is never possible to eliminate all risk from giving birth or from being alive. But it is up to you, the pregnant woman, to inform yourself, weigh the risks, and make a responsible decision based on minimizing risk and maximizing satisfaction for you and your family. This book is intended to help you to focus your ideas and come to a decision that best expresses your real feelings and attitudes.

HOSPITAL OPTIONS

Hospital birth has changed a great deal in the past ten years. The homebirth movement and the increase in

---

[19]For more information see Ina May Gaskin, *Spiritual Midwifery* (Summertown, TN: The Book Publishing Company, 1978), pp. 474–5.

---

[20]"Statement on Home Delivery," American College of Obstetricians and Gynecologists, March 1979.

---

[21]Hinds, et al, "Neonatal Outcome in Planned v. Unplanned Out-of-Hospital Birth in Kentucky," JAMA, Vol. 253, No. 11, March 15, 1985. And Burnett, et al, "Home Delivery and Neonatal Mortality in North Carolina," JAMA, 244:2741-45, 1980.

free-standing birth centers, together with a declining birth rate and rising costs, have caused many hospitals to add birthing rooms as an option to attract couples. While a "home-like atmosphere" will never replace the advantages of giving birth at home, the added security of having hospital resources so close by is a plus for many couples.

Birth centers are both revolutionizing hospital birth and providing a much more human and humane birth for thousands of couples who would never consider having their baby at home. And hospitals must continue changing because of the inconsistency between birth-center and standard procedures. Why can a woman in one room birth wearing her own nightgown in the labor bed with her family around her, without a shave, enema, IV or fetal monitor, while her equally low-risk sister a few doors away is flat on her back with her legs in stirrups, draped with sterile sheets on a narrow delivery table and wired to a glucose drip and an electronic fetal monitor? Women need to reclaim birth as their own and to ask for, and insist on being treated with, respect for themselves and the birthing process. Hospitals today will comply with women's demands due to economics, if nothing else. There is no longer scientific justification for most standard hospital procedures. In fact, follow-up studies of birth-center deliveries have clearly shown the superiority of fewer interventive approaches.[22]

If you are contemplating a hospital birth, make sure to shop around for hospitals and doctors who will give you the kind of birth you want. Don't feel trapped by your insurance! You should be able to avoid standard "prepping" (pubic shave and enema), have no IV or fetal monitor unless an emergency arises, be free to labor and deliver in whatever position you choose, have the baby with you continuously after the birth and sign out for early dismissal if you want. Talk with your doctor or midwife and formulate a birth plan in writing that can be available to remind your doctor of his commitments and to advise hospital staff of your wishes.[23]

If you are going to give birth in a birthing room or birth center, be advised that the procedure and techniques of your attendant make a far greater difference than the decor of the room or the inclusion of an expensive birthing chair. If you are giving birth with midwives, you have a much greater possibility of a normal birth. But sometimes they, too, are bound by protocols and fear of how their statistics will look to hospital staff, so they may not have as much patience as a midwife in another setting. Interview your doctor or midwife and ask what percentage of his or her clients deliver with a cesarean, episiotomy, fetal monitor, and so forth. Ask specific questions to avoid answers such as "We only do that when necessary" (but he neglects to tell you that it's "necessary" 25% or 95% of the time!).

If you are planning on using a birthing room, investigate what the protocols are, so you don't suddenly find yourself "risked out" and relegated to a standard hospital delivery for an unexpected variation from the norm. And what if the birthing room is occupied when you go into labor? Do your investigating in advance to lessen the number of surprises when you are in labor.

YOUR OWN BIRTH DECISION

You need to make the decision that is right for *you.* Sometimes you have to work hard to create the options you want, while other times it is hard to find clarity within yourself or agreement from your partner. If you are undecided about where you want to give birth, the exercises in *Pregnant Feelings* can help to clarify what is important to you and help you achieve it. If you are planning a vaginal birth after a cesarean, you will benefit by the invaluable support from *Silent Knife: Cesarean Prevention and Vaginal Birth after Cesarean* by Cohen and Estner.[24]

Whatever your choice, studying the process of birth will be invaluable for you. Even if you prefer a homebirth but end up with a hospital delivery, your having informed yourself will ensure a hospital experience quite different from that of someone who has abnegated responsibility for the birth process.

This book is designed as a practical guide for pregnancy and homebirth. At the end of most chapters is a list of other books which explore in detail the issues involved in making the homebirth decision, give personal accounts of home deliveries, and so forth. Read! Confidence based on knowledge and certainty is one of the keys to a satisfying homebirth experience.

Talk with other couples. If there are homebirth classes in your area, be sure to attend them; no book can replace the first-hand information and emotional support they provide. Chapter 4 lists the national organizations providing such classes. If there are no classes specifically geared for homebirth couples in your area, you can benefit from the Informed Homebirth cassette tape course of twelve lessons that supplement this book.

Above all, communicate with each other as a couple. If your partner is apprehensive about homebirth, really listening to his fears, discussing birth, reading

[22]See "Birthing Renaissance" in *Pregnant Feelings* by Rahima Baldwin and Terra Palmarini (Berkeley, CA: Celestial Arts, 1986).

[23]*Pregnant Feelings* also has detailed information on interviewing doctors and forming a birth plan.

[24]Nancy Cohen and Lois Estner. *Silent Knife* (South Hadley, MA: Bergin & Garvey, 1983).

and talking with other people will often help him to see things differently. After all, men in our culture are given very little support for being in touch with their bodies, and practically no information or feeling for their relationship to the normal birth process.

If, on the other hand, it is the man who is pushing for a home delivery, he should recognize that the ultimate decision needs to be his wife's. My experience has been that if a woman wants to give birth in a hospital, she will probably end up there one way or another. It is important for a homebirth that the couple be in agreement about what they are doing and have a high level of intention and responsibility.

Once you have made your decision to have a homebirth, there is still a great deal to do. Later chapters in this book discuss the issues of finding prenatal care, finding a midwife and preparing an emergency backup plan. The sooner these activities get underway, the better, especially if you live in an area without much support for homebirth.

Because we have all been culturally conditioned with so many irrational attitudes about birth, you may well encounter opposition to your plans at some point, whether from friends, family, doctors, or other members of the medical community whom you approach for health care. It is best not to argue with people if it fosters upset. Instead, focus your attention on building a community of support to help your intention strengthen and grow; you are not alone in your knowledge and convictions. If you encounter people who are worried but truly open-minded, recommend that they read some of the books on the subject.

We are living in a time of rapid change in our culture's attitudes about birth. You are part of that change. Our right to give birth as we choose is a right well worth reclaiming.

FOR FURTHER READING

A Good Birth, A Safe Birth by Diana Korte and Roberta Scaer. How to get the options you want within a hospital setting.

Homebirth by Sheila Kitzinger. Advantages and risks of home birth, with both statistical information and personal accounts by women who have chosen this alternative. Kitzinger is a British childbirth educator and anthropologist who had her five daughters at home.

Birth Reborn by Dr. Michel Odent. A look at what women-centered birth with midwives is like at Odent's clinic in France. Excellent book!

Birthrights by Sally Inch. What every parent should know about giving birth in hospitals.

Five Standards for Safe Childbearing by David Stewart. An extremely comprehensive review of the statistics for midwifery and home births. Supports the five standards of good nutrition, skillful midwifery, natural childbirth, birth at home and breastfeeding.

Giving Birth: Alternatives in Childbirth by Barbara Katz Rothman. Analyzes current obstetrical practice as compared to midwifery practices and how sexism affects it all. Formerly called: *In Labor: Women and Power in the Birth Place.*

Immaculate Deception by Suzanne Arms. An in-depth presentation of the way in which American hospital practices are robbing women of their birth experience; contrasts with birth in European countries.

Informed Homebirth Tape Series by Rahima Baldwin. Twelve lessons on six cassettes that supplement this book. From Informed Homebirth, Box 3675, Ann Arbor, MI 48106.

Lying In: A History of Childbirth in America by Richard and Dorothy Wertz. A fascinating study of childbirth practices from colonial times to the present.

Open Season: A Survival Guide for Natural Childbirth and VBAC in the 90s by Nancy Wainer Cohen. A rallying cry and wakeup call for anyone interested in natural birth.

Pregnant Feelings by Rahima Baldwin and Terra Palmarini. Includes practical ways to clarify your emotions and values to create the kind of birth you want.

Silent Knife: Cesarean Prevention and Vaginal Birth after Cesarean by Nancy Cohen and Lois Estner. A must, given this nation's cesarean rate! Well-documented, preventative and very practical.

Special Delivery video by Rahima Baldwin. This video shows birth in various settings, emphasizes choices and psychological aspects. From IBP, P.O. Box 3675, Ann Arbor, MI 48106.

Spiritual Midwifery by Ina May Gaskin. Contains classic birthing tales from members of The Farm, an intentional community in Tennessee where births are assisted by midwives. Excellent section on birth and midwifery with a great deal of practical advice.

WHY I CHOSE A HOMEBIRTH

Sheila Sabine

I had my child at home because I wanted to have complete control over the quality of my birth experience. I wanted rituals, fresh flowers, candles and loved ones surrounding me to share in this dance of my womanhood. I couldn't imagine leaving my nest during labor and driving to a hospital when all my instincts grounded me to my own private space.

I had danced throughout my pregnancy and had confidence that my body, mind and spirit were prepared to meet the challenge of labor and birth. Most important, I really believed that a homebirth would provide a safer environment for both me and my child. My beliefs were based on reading, talking with friends, and seeing a hospital birth. All those "what ifs" poking me in all directions allowed me to get clear about my own strengths and weaknesses.

I thought about the birth I had seen in a small hut on the Mexican coast, where lovely Carmen delivered her tenth child quietly in the night as her other children slept around her in the same room. I thought of my friend, Ellen, and her courage and births in a cabin in Gold Hill. Images of my great-grandmother and all the women of the world floated around my round belly. Their babies were born on this planet—beautiful, alive, healthy beings—born simply and naturally, without the assistance of technologically advanced tools and medication.

Mara Sabine Link was born on March 28, amidst flowers, candles and friends. My womanhood blossomed its fullest to meet this new being. Although a doctor was present, the choices were my own. The responsibility was my own. The quality of the experience was as I intended it to be—perfect.

WHY I CHOSE A HOSPITAL BIRTH

Celie Tucker-Lansing

My preparation for TenEyck's birth became an integration of all aspects of my life. When I found out I was pregnant, I started taking prenatal exercise classes and joined a midwifery study group.

I began to see how complex the birthing process can be, and I wondered whether I would have my baby at home or in the hospital. I was with a close friend during her wonderful hospital birth and close to another who had planned a homebirth but ended with a very uncomfortable hospital birth. As I heard of many subsequent births I realized how subjective the experience is. I felt that people were setting up expectations for the birth that were much too idealistic. These expectations seemed to set people up only to be let down. For instance, if the parents were particularly attached to having a homebirth, they seemed to have a negative experience if for any reason they had to go to the hospital. So I decided to entertain all possible fantasies of what the birth would be like, and to gather all the tools necessary to facilitate anything that might happen. I started Informed Homebirth classes without having formed a particular attachment to either a home or hospital birth.

After the first class, which Yates and I both found very informative, we saw our doctor, Julie Carpenter. Our talk with her was probably a major deciding factor. She felt that it was best to have a first baby in the hospital. We asked how much time we would have in an emergency situation. She said as little as seconds, but usually seven minutes. We live thirty minutes from town. My feeling after our conversation was that I wanted the safest possible birth. This is not necessarily a hospital birth, but in Boulder a homebirth is without a doctor, which was important to me. The atmosphere was also important to me, but that was my need and might not be the baby's need. Also I had come to know that Julie was very accommodating of individual needs and desires, and I felt good about what could happen in the hospital atmosphere with her.

I continued to take the Informed Homebirth classes as I felt comfortable in knowing I could handle a homebirth if necessary. Yates stopped going, but I was still sharing the information with him. I realized while taking the classes the most responsible person in the homebirth situation is the partner, who needs to have as much information concerning a birth as possible and to feel comfortable making a decision in an emergency sit-

situation. I cannot stress this enough. Yates felt queasy at the sight of blood and didn't feel he wanted that much responsibility concerning the life of his child. He was very emotionally involved with our baby coming. I felt his emotions could be overwhelming for him and make it difficult for him to make a decision in an emergency, although I trust him ultimately.

While taking the homebirth classes, I began teaching a prenatal class offering exercise and massage. This became a great support system for all of us involved. My classes helped me to integrate all that I had learned and prepare me for TenEyck's birth in a much clearer and more meaningful way.

Toward the end of my pregnancy Yates and I took a prepared childbirth class through the hospital   If it had been the only class we had taken I would have felt very out of touch with the birthing. The material just wasn't extensive enough for my needs. Yates found the class amusing and wasn't able to take it seriously. It seemed too mundane and didn't offer enough helpful hints.

TenEyck was born a week early. I had begun to dilate two weeks before his birth and was already three centimeters dilated. Braxton-Hicks contractions were frequent but not painful. I was on the couch at 8:00 A.M. the morning of his birth talking with my sister, Melanie. I told her I was having contractions, but wasn't sure if this was it. Melanie was rubbing my back as I was squatting. I felt a snap inside and then a trickle. I was still not sure. My mother came downstairs, took in the situation and said, "Let's call the doctor just to be in touch."

Julie said to come to a friend's house in town. We left about 9:15 in a camper that was wonderfully padded with sleeping bags and foam pads. Melanie was doing touch relaxation with me, touching areas that were tense, while Yates was breathing with me. I moved around to find a comfortable position. My contractions were intense but not as painful as I had imagined. My focus was on remaining relaxed. On the way down I told Susan, who was driving, to go straight to the hospital. She backed the camper into emergency. I waited for a contraction to pass, crawled out onto the stretcher, and while being wheeled up to OB thought I was going to defecate all over the stretcher, and panted.

In the labor room the nurse checked my cervix, said I was ten centimeters, went to call Julie and returned. I asked her to check the baby's heartbeat. She did so cheerfully as if in my employ—which of course she was.

They wheeled me into the delivery room after they got in touch with Julie. One nurse told another that Julie had said not to use stirrups. Julie was willing to let me explore positions on the delivery table. As it turned out I ended up in the typical hospital delivery position; but with my mother and the nurse holding my legs, which provided much more support with the warmth of contact.

The lights were low, and I had all the people I wanted with me, even though it was bending the rules a bit. It was great to have such a team. TenEyck's head was visible all this time. We got into position, then worked with the contractions, stretching the perineum to avoid an episiotomy. Julie massaged the perineum and I pushed, then relaxed, then pushed and held, panting with small exhalations so as not to release pressure. Everyone was involved, rooting me on, until finally TenEyck burst upon the scene all in one contraction at 10:52 A.M. Melanie and a friend, Cheryl, both exclaimed, "It's a boy!" Julie shushed them as TenEyck was suctioned, then laid on my belly. His skin was like velvet. I melted to his touch. We were all in tears. Yates had wanted a son. It was all magic to me.

I delivered the placenta, had one stitch and was being massaged to contract my uterus. I wasn't contracting as much as Julie wanted, so she asked if I would take a shot of pitocin. I asked everything that I needed to know about it, and told her to go ahead. I breathed with the strong pressure to extract any clots. It was much less painful.

TenEyck was then given a LeBoyer bath. He floated in the water easily and looked around. His presence was so full and his perception wide open, it was incredible.

Yates then carried him into the nursery where only the most necessary procedures were done: He was weighed and measured, given the eye drops required by law, and given vitamin K (which I take myself).

I was in my room now and Yates carried TenEyck in. Julie helped him to take the breast and he nursed and fell asleep. Yates held him until we checked out that afternoon. All I could say to Julie was that it seemed so easy. She said, "It's you. Many people have it a lot harder." I felt at that moment that all my work had been brought to bear.

TenEyck is a very content little person and has made it fun to be a mother. I love it. I'm still teaching prenatal classes, and have started a mothers-and-babies class in which we do baby massage and exercise, teach parenting skills and exchange ideas and experience. I still work to understand how to accommodate both our needs, but TenEyck is part of the work I've developed for myself, and I feel complete.

CHAPTER TWO

Prenatal Care

THE IMPORTANCE OF PRENATAL CARE

The most crucial factors in determining birth outcomes all happen before labor begins: prenatal care, nutrition and training for childbirth. Prenatal care is crucial for every birth, but it is especially vital for homebirths. When you go into labor at home, you need to know that you and the baby are in good health, that you are not anemic, that the baby is head down, and so forth.

Prenatal care fulfills two functions. The first is screening, that is, determining which couples are good candidates for homebirth and which births should *not* take place at home. Prenatal care can detect or predict about 80 to 85 percent of all high-risk pregnancies, and 90 to 95 percent of low-risk prepared births proceed without incident. Those women having risk factors prior to pregnancy or developing problems before labor begins can investigate hospital or birth center alternatives which will allow for their safest and best delivery.

The other function of prenatal care is to allow potential or actual problems to be diagnosed and handled before labor begins. If, for example, a blood test reveals low iron, iron supplements can be taken to bring the hematocrit level up to normal before the birth. If you are contemplating a homebirth, you want to know that you are entering it with you and your baby in the best possible condition.

FINDING PRENATAL CARE

There are three ways to receive prenatal care: from a doctor, from a clinic, or from a midwife. Each has its advantages and disadvantages.

If your homebirth will be attended by a doctor, of course that doctor will also provide prenatal care. But even if your birth attendant will not be a doctor it can be useful to have prenatal care with a sympathetic M.D., because he or she may be willing to meet you at the hospital if medical attention becomes necessary. (This is more likely after the doctor gets to know you and finds out that you are informed and being responsible about your decision.) Unfortunately, it is within a doctor's rights to refuse you prenatal care if he knows that you are planning a homebirth, or to offer prenatal care only in conjunction with a delivery fee. Out of fear of malpractice such doctors only add to the problem they are trying to avoid.

Therefore, you may have to do some investigating to find a sympathetic doctor. Check with friends, La Leche League leaders or prepared childbirth teachers. You can get their numbers through hospitals, doctors' offices and the Red Cross. Osteopaths (and, in some states, chiropractors) are licensed to do births and are often more open to homebirth than M.D.s.

Clinics offer prenatal care, usually at a much lower cost than a doctor. This also will register you for the hospital, should you need to go. Their disadvantages tend to include long waits and not knowing which doctor you will see. Don't forget to investigate osteopathic hospitals and clinics in your area.

If your midwife offers her own prenatal care, it can be a good chance to get to know her better before the birth. She will probably ask you to go to a clinic to have laboratory work done early in pregnancy. If she doesn't do her own care, she should go over your records during visits with you.

TAKING RESPONSIBILITY

We are used to a medical system in which doctors maintain their knowledge in secret, even to the extent of writing instructions to pharmacists in Latin abbreviations! However, in prenatal care (or any other care for that matter) we are concerned with our own health and are paying for the work to be done, and we have a right to know the outcome. You should arrange with your doctor or clinic to give you a copy of all prenatal records, including lab results. In this chapter we will discuss what prenatal care includes and what the results mean, so you will be able to interpret them. Know your own body, and take responsibility for it! Don't leave it in someone else's hands, no matter how well-meaning they are.

YOUR PRENATAL CARE

Prenatal care is usually begun in the third month of pregnancy. Most prenatal clinics ask you to come in once a month until the eighth month, then every two weeks or every week as you approach your due date.

A thorough medical history should be taken during your initial visit to give a picture of your menstrual history, methods of birth control, past pregnancies or abortions, important illnesses, surgery, medications or drugs. Your family's health history should be noted to see if there is a tendency towards diabetes or hypertension.

Now refer to the charts beginning on p. 23, which you can keep yourself (or you can request a xerox of your doctor's records). Keeping a copy of your health records is important, not only for your own information, but because you may not have continuity of health care prenatally, at the birth, and in case of any difficulties requiring hospitalization. Ask for an explanation of anything you don't understand. Good communication is important at every stage of the process. Write down any questions you have about your pregnancy so you don't forget to ask them.

PELVIC EXAMINATION AND ASSESSMENT

Early in pregnancy a pelvic exam may be done to confirm pregnancy. The uterus is palpated, and a softening of the cervix as well as a change in color signal pregnancy. Vaginal exams are not usually done again until the last month, to check the position of the baby and the condition of the cervix, and to look for active genital herpes, a viral infection usually requiring a cesarean.

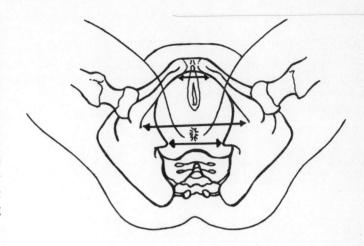

FIGURE 2-1. *Measuring the pelvis.*

At some point, assessment of the pelvic bones will be done to see how big your pelvis is (Figure 2-1). A fist is placed externally between your ischial tuberosities ("sit-bones"); the pubic arch is felt in front to see if it is wide or narrow; the "diagonal conjugate" is felt vaginally from the pubic bone to the sacrum, and the distance between the ischial spines is felt.

Pelvimetry by hand, X-ray or ultrasound only gives an impression of pelvic shape. It does not tell how much your pelvic bones will stretch when the ligaments relax during labor, how strong your contractions will be, and how much the baby's head will become smaller by molding. Pelvimetry is worse than useless if remarks like "a narrow arch" or "prominent spines" undermine your confidence. Don't let any medical approximations lessen your conviction that your body is ideally suited for giving birth!

TOXEMIA

One of the main things checked for each visit is signs of toxemia (pre-eclampsia/eclampsia), which manifests by swelling of the hands, feet and face (edema), sudden weight gain, protein in the urine and high blood pressure. If unrecognized, toxemia can lead to headaches, dizziness, coma, stillbirth and maternal death.

Dr. Tom Brewer, in his twelve-year project working with high-risk mothers in Contra Costa County, California, has shown that toxemia is a result of malnutrition, sometimes from low socio-economic conditions or even from the low-calorie, low-salt diets often prescribed by doctors in an attempt to counteract one of the symptoms of toxemia! Slight edema, or swelling, can be normal during pregnancy. Read the next chapter on nutrition, and if you have enough trouble with any of the symptoms to warrant concern, read *What Every Pregnant Woman Should Know: The Truth About Diets and Drugs in Pregnancy*, by Gail Sforza Brewer with Tom Brewer, M.D.

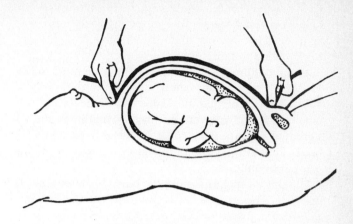

FIGURE 2-4. *Measuring the growth of the uterus.*

FETAL GROWTH AND DEVELOPMENT

It is important to determine how your baby is growing. Knowing due dates helps assess pre- and post-maturity. Watching development helps detect light-for-dates (low birth weight) babies, twins, and hydramnios (excessive amniotic fluid), among other things.

If you have regular menstrual periods and know when your last one was, you can calculate your approximate due date by taking the date of the first day of your last menstrual period (for example, June 15), subtracting three months and adding seven days (March 22, in this example). Your expected due date is 280 days from the first day of your last period (as above), even though you conceived about two weeks later and the *gestational age* of your baby at term is only about 266 days.

If your period is irregular (after breastfeeding or using the pill, for example) or if you were pregnant and had enough spotting the first month to think it was a period, your dates may be off and you may need to reassess the baby's age as the pregnancy progresses.

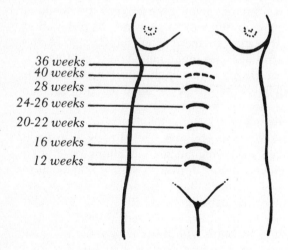

36 weeks
40 weeks
28 weeks
24-26 weeks
20-22 weeks
16 weeks
12 weeks

FIGURE 2-3. *Height of the uterus by weeks.*

Normal uterine growth is measured each visit by noting the size of the uterus from the pubic bone to the *fundus*, or top (Figures 2-3 and 2-4). Reporting when you first feel the baby move (usually around 16 to 18 weeks, although sometimes earlier with second or subse-

quent babies) can also help determine the baby's development. The baby's heartbeat can first be heard around 16 to 18 weeks with a normal stethoscope or fetoscope (earlier with a Doptone) and should be heard by twenty weeks.

WHAT IS CHECKED EACH VISIT

Weight: A gain of 25–35 pounds is healthy during pregnancy. The important thing is *what* you are eating, and that it include sufficient protein, vitamins and minerals.

Edema: Water retention and some swelling of the ankles, hands or feet occurs in 80 to 90 percent of pregnancies. See earlier discussion on toxemia.

Blood Pressure: The mythical normal is 120/80 (systolic, or pumping, pressure/diastolic, or released, pressure). Know what your normal range is.

Urinalysis: Urine is checked with a dipstick for ketones, protein and glucose. *Ketones* are a by-product of fat metabolism (you're not eating adequately if you're losing weight!). *Protein* is an early sign of toxemia (increase your protein intake and reevaluate your nutrition); it can also be a by-product of urinary-tract infection or some kidney infections if you are eating 80–100 grams of protein a day. *Sugar* can be a sign of prediabetes. Again, reevaluate your eating habits and eliminate sugars, soft drinks and anything else that is contributing to the condition. Get it under control!

Ask your doctor or midwife if she wants a urine sample from first thing in the morning and if she wants a "clean catch" (mid-stream) to examine for microbes.

Height of the Fundus: The uterus is measured from the pubic bone to the fundus (top) from about the twentieth week on. Between 20 and 36 weeks, growth is about 1 cm per week, and the number approximately equals the number of weeks' gestation.

Palpation and Fetal Heart Tones: The heart tones will be listened for starting about the sixteenth to eighteenth week with a stethoscope or a fetoscope, or even earlier with a Doptone, an ultrasonic device which magnifies the sounds so everyone can hear them. Normal range is 120–160 beats per minute. Listen to it in the doctor's office; then try having your partner listen at home with a stethoscope (an empty toilet paper roll often works well). Time it for 15 seconds and multiply by 4 for the rate per minute.

Palpation means feeling the baby to determine its position. This is especially important in the last few months and just before delivery. Again, learn from your prenatal visits so you and your partner can try it at home.

LABORATORY WORK

Complete lab work is done once, early in pregnancy. The hematocrit or hemoglobin count is often repeated around the eighth month to make sure you are not anemic. The gonorrhea culture is often done in the last month, as is the vag strep culture.

All blood work is done from a single sample taken from a vein in the arm, except the hematocrit, which is done by pricking the finger. If your hematocrit is low, you should request that it be redone from a vein in your hand, which often yields a higher and more accurate figure.

VDRL: Wasserman bloodtest for syphilis, which the baby can contract. A false positive is sometimes possible.

Rh: Analysis of the blood to determine if the mother is Rh^+ or Rh^-. If Rh^-, the Rh/or Coomb's titer test should be done around 20 weeks and again at 32 weeks to see if sensitization and antibody production have occurred.

Blood Type: To have in case emergency blood is needed.

Rubella: Analysis of the blood to determine if the mother is immune to rubella (measles); if not, she should be especially careful to avoid exposure during pregnancy and might want to consider being inoculated immediately after the baby is born to prevent the possibility of exposure in later pregnancies.

Hematocrit (Hct): Analysis of the blood to determine anemia. If below 37 percent, it is usually repeated at each visit until you raise it through eating foods rich in iron, taking iron supplements, etc. Percentage considered anemic varies with altitude.

Hemoglobin Count: Sometimes done instead of the hematocrit. It is approximately equal to one third the hematocrit number. A count of 12.6 is recommended for homebirth—check with your attendant.

THE RH FACTOR

The Rh factor is a substance found on the surface of red blood cells. Most people have this factor and are thus "Rh positive" (Rh^+). If you are among the 15 percent with Rh^- blood and the father is Rh^+, your baby can be either positive or negative. When the baby is Rh^+, a special situation arises.

If any Rh^+ blood enters your bloodstream (through abortions, miscarriages, blood transfusions, etc.) your body reacts to the positive blood cells as foreign and produces antibodies against them. This is the state of being *immunized* or *sensitized,* and this is what the titer test is used to detect.

If this is your first pregnancy and/or your titer tests show no sensitization, the baby is usually not in any danger, since sensitization almost always occurs when the placenta separates, which is too late to affect this baby. This sensitization, which would endanger future babies, can be prevented by making sure you have an injection of Rhogam within 72 hours after the birth of an Rh *positive* baby (take some of the cord blood in a test tube to determine the baby's Rh factor).

Rhogam keeps you from producing your own permanent Rh antibodies and prevents your blood from recognizing the baby's blood cells as "foreign." In this way, it prevents the production of antibodies so there won't be danger to the baby in your next pregnancy. You should have a shot of Rhogam after each abortion, miscarriage or delivery of an Rh^+ baby to prevent the possibility of Rh hemolytic disease in future pregnancies.

If you are Rh^- and are already sensitized through past pregnancies, abortions or miscarriages, you should deliver in the hospital because there is a danger that these antibodies can pass into the bloodstream of an Rh^+ fetus and start destroying the baby's Rh^+ red blood cells. The result is Rh hemolytic disease, which can cause anemia, heart failure, brain damage or death. In some babies it shows up *in utero;* in others it is characterized by jaundice (yellowness of the skin) in the *first 24 hours* and usually requires a transfusion and other intensive care measures.

HIV & HBV: Most healthcare providers will want to see if you have been exposed to HIV (precursor of AIDS) or hepatitis B virus.

Tine Test: A test on the forearm for tuberculosis. If the place of injection turns red in forty-eight hours, further testing should be done. If there is no reaction, the test is negative.

Pap: A pap smear is done annually (and often at the time of initial prenatal visits) to detect cervical cancer.

Urinalysis, micro and urine culture: A further examination and culturing of the urine is done if a urinary infection is suspected.

Gonorrhea Culture (GC): A swab is taken from the cervix and cultured to detect gonorrhea, which can infect the baby and cause blindness immediately after birth. Only about 80 percent effective in detecting gonorrhea in women.

PALPATION AND FETAL HEART TONES

You can palpate or feel the position of the baby yourself. This puts you in more direct relationship with both the baby and your own body. It is also good to work together with your partner, both feeling the various parts of the baby. The following instructions are as if someone is examining you, but you can do these things yourself. Also add your own internal data to the process: Where have you been feeling kicking lately? Have you felt a lot of body movement? Where do you feel the greatest mass of the baby? And next time your birth attendant palpates the position, ask to feel the baby, too.

Prepare yourself by first emptying your bladder. Then lie down in a comfortable position with your knees slightly elevated, or sit back propped up with pillows, since it can hinder circulation for you to lie flat on your back for too long.

First: stand or kneel by the mother's side and feel above the pubic bone with the thumb and fingers of one hand (Figure 2-5). During the last month of pregnancy, the head will be down in 90 percent of cases, but don't jump to conclusions! The head will feel harder, smoother, rounder than the buttocks. If it is the head, it will be easier to move from side to side (if not engaged in the pelvis), and the body will not move with it. It is often possible to feel the groove of the neck as the head is moved.

Next try to locate the back and the baby's arms and legs. Go in fairly deeply with the sides of both hands, pushing with one toward the other (Figure 2-6). The back feels firmer and smoother, offering even resistance along a curve. The small parts feel knobbly and correspond to where the mother feels movement. It may be difficult to feel the back if the baby is in a posterior position or if there is lots of fluid.

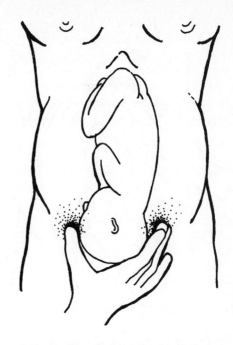

FIGURE 2-5. *Feeling the lower pole of the uterus.*

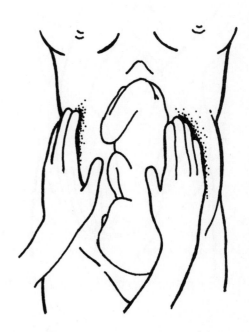

FIGURE 2-6. *Palpating the sides.*

Now feel the top of the uterus (Figure 2-7). If you are feeling the breech (buttocks), it will be felt as less definite, softer, more irregular, less round and not as mobile as the head. The feet should be felt nearby. The breech is felt as being continuous with the back, without a groove as with the neck. When it is moved from side to side, the body moves as well.

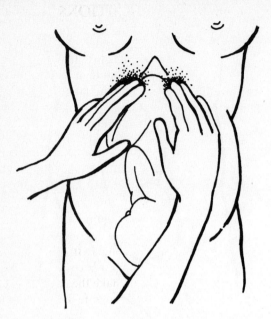

FIGURE 2-7. *Feeling the top of the uterus.*

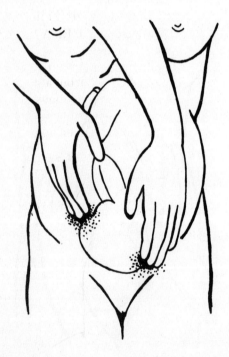

FIGURE 2-8. *Checking for flexion of the head.*

Move your fingers down the sides of the uterus towards the pubic bone. Notice which hand encounters a prominent spot first (Figure 2-8). If the head is well flexed, it should be on the opposite side from the back. Continue down until you reach the pubic bone. If your fingers move outward as they reach the bone, the head is probably engaged (also check by trying to move the head from side to side—it won't move if it's engaged (Figure

2-9). If you can feel your fingers coming together around the baby's head before you reach the pubic bone, the head is probably not engaged.

Palpation can be difficult if the abdominal walls are particularly strong, if there is a layer of fat over the abdomen, or if there is a great deal of fluid. Make sure the mother is relaxed, with knees slightly bent. Have her breathe! Make sure your hands are warm, and use a loving touch. Press quite firmly, and take your time.

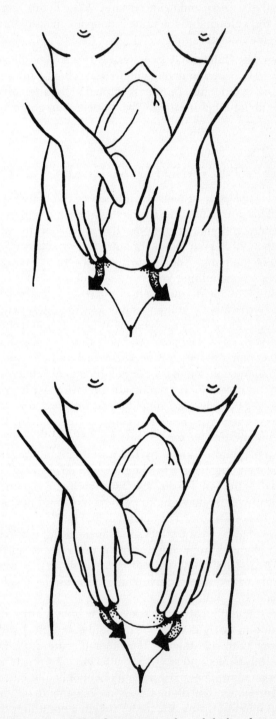

FIGURE 2-9. *(a) Head not engaged, and (b) head engaged.*

CHANGING A BREECH POSITION

Many babies are breech early in pregnancy, but about two-thirds turn spontaneously to a vertex presentation, leaving about 3 to 4 percent of babies breech at term.

If your baby is in a head-up position in the eighth month, there is a simple exercise you can do to help it turn.

Twice a day, with an empty stomach, lie on your back on the floor for ten minutes with about three pillows under your bottom and none under your head. Your pelvis should be raised about 9 to 12 inches, knees bent and feet on the floor

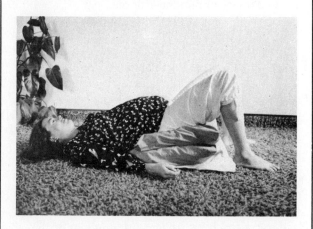

FIGURE 2-10. *Position for turning a breech baby.*

Dr. Juliet M. DeSa Souza, who developed this exercise, reported that in 1000 cases studied the success rate using this exercise was 89 percent overall, and 96 percent in her private practice.

The exercise should be done twice a day from the thirtieth week until the baby turns head down (usually 2–3 weeks), then discontinued. Even if this fails to work, it makes it easier to do external version (using the hands on the abdomen to turn the baby). Many doctors are reluctant to do external version, but some midwives are having good success with it.[1]

---

[1]For further information on external version, see Ina May Gaskin, *Spiritual Midwifery* (Summertown, TN: The Book Publishing Co., 1978), pp. 337–9.

DeSa Souza's study reported in *VII World Congress of Gynecology and Obstetrics*, October, 1976. (Princeton, N.J.: Excerpta Medica), p. 121.

UNUSUAL POSITIONS

It is important to have an accurate assessment of the baby's position before labor begins. If it has been a while since your last examination or if you have felt a great deal of movement since your last prenatal visit, the position should be reassessed.

Once the head is down, in the eighth month or so, it tends to stay down because of gravity and the decreasing space in which the baby can move about. But babies have been known to turn just before labor, so stay alert.

Knowing about a posterior position can help you know what to expect in labor. For example, if the back of the baby's head is pressing against your backbone ("back labor"), you will feel more discomfort and lower back pain, and labor may be longer. If you discover a transverse lie (baby crosswise) or a breech presentation (buttocks or feet first), you can make the necessary decisions in advance to provide for the safe delivery of your baby.

LISTENING FOR THE FETAL HEART BEAT

The heartbeat is probably easiest to hear using a fetoscope (Figures 2-11 and 2-12), but a stethoscope will also often work. In either case, you must use bare skin and press quite firmly to pick up the heart tones, which sound something like a watch ticking under a pillow.

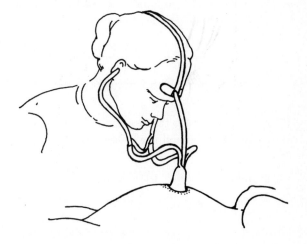

FIGURE 2-11. *Listening for fetal heart tones with a fetoscope.*

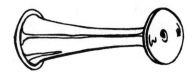

FIGURE 2-12. *Pinard's (horn) fetoscope.*

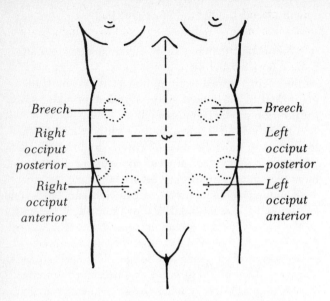

Breech
Right occiput posterior
Right occiput anterior
Breech
Left occiput posterior
Left occiput anterior

FIGURE 2-13. *Where you might hear the baby's heart with various positions.*

When the baby's head is flexed, the heartbeat is transmitted through the back of the shoulder. It will therefore be heard loudest over the place on the abdomen that is closest to the back. In the most common position, left occiput anterior, the heart tones are usually heard in the lower left quadrant of the belly. But try various spots (Figure 2-13). Heart tones can usually be heard after the eighteenth or twentieth week of pregnancy. You are listening for a very fast and regular beat, between 120 and 160 beats per minute. Once you have located it, count the number of beats in 15 seconds and multiply by 4 to get the beats per minute.

FACTORS INCREASING THE RISK FOR HOMEBIRTH

If you have any of the following conditions, a home delivery is medically contraindicated.

FACTORS RELATED TO THE MOTHER'S HEALTH

Poor nutrition, poor health, lack of vitality, very overweight or underweight.
Diabetes mellitus
Hypertension (high blood pressure)
Heart disease
Kidney disease
Active genital herpes at the time of birth—necessitates a c-section as the baby can contract it and develop brain damage or blindness, or die.

FACTORS RELATED TO PREVIOUS PREGNANCIES

Previous cesarean section—we know of no doctor who would condone a home delivery for a vaginal birth after cesarean, but an increasing number of VBAC mothers are delivering at home. See *Silent Knife* by Cohen and Estner for real and imagined risk of uterine rupture.
Previous stillbirth—unless the cause is known and not likely to repeat.
Hard-to-control hemorrhage with previous birth— likely to repeat.

DANGER SIGNS OF PREGNANCY

Consult with your birth attendant immediately if you experience any of the following:

ANY BLEEDING FROM THE VAGINA

In the first trimester, this can be a sign of possible spontaneous abortion; in the second or third trimester it can have non-placental causes, but is one of the signs of low-lying placenta (placenta praevia) or of the placenta separating from the uterus (abruptio placenta).

SEVERE, PERSISTENT ABDOMINAL PAIN

Can be a sign of an extra-uterine pregnancy, abruptio placenta, appendicitis, etc.

SEVERE HEADACHES IN THE LAST THREE MONTHS OR DIM OR BLURRY VISION

These are signs associated with advanced toxemia.

NO FETAL MOVEMENT FOR 24 HOURS AFTER THE FIFTH MONTH

If you feel there is something wrong, have it checked out.

PREMATURE RUPTURE OF THE MEMBRANES

Once the waters rupture, you and the baby are open to infection. Labor may result, or you may need antibiotics and induced labor. Occasionally, the water bag will leak, then reseal and stay sealed for weeks, but this should be under close observation because of the risk of infection.

FACTORS RELATED TO THIS PREGNANCY

Anemia—can lead to shock from blood loss, fetal distress, weakness and infection. Be aware of false anemia of late pregnancy.

Toxemia—can result in stillbirth, seizures, coma and death.

Rh⁻ mother with antibody sensitization—baby's red blood cells can be attacked, resulting in anemia, heart failure, brain damage or death; might necessitate blood transfusions, or can cause stillbirth.

Polyhydramnios (too much amniotic fluid)—greater risk of malpresentation, cord prolapse and hemorrhage. Birth defects in the baby in one-third of cases.

Bleeding beyond twenty weeks, especially in the last trimester—possible placenta praevia or abruptio placenta.

Multiple Pregnancy—danger to the second twin is greater; often one is breech; prematurity and respiratory distress syndrome common; postpartum hemorrhage more likely through distended uterus.

Breech presentation (buttocks first)—danger to the baby is greater: see emergency section on breech. Never attempt a breech at home except with someone who has good experience delivering breech babies and who has good backup.

Cephalo-pelvic disproportion—get a second opinion, since it's hard to predict strength of contractions and how much the head will mold until you are in labor.

Premature rupture of the membranes—notify your birth attendant; both mother and baby are open to infection once the waters break, but avoiding vaginal exams decreases the risk.

Labor begins more than three weeks before known due date—dangers of prematurity include greater trauma to the baby, increased stillbirth rate, more prone to cold stress, hyaline membrane disease and other respiratory problems.

Labor begins more than two weeks late—have an estriol check to see if your placenta is still functioning well. If not, labor may need to be induced. Post-maturity has a high stillborn rate, too; longer and more traumatic labor because the head is larger and more calcified.

OTHER FACTORS WHICH INCREASE THE RISK

Age: under 16 or over 35 for a first baby, or over 40 for any pregnancy—statistically more problems. However, an older woman could successfully give birth at home, depending on her health, nutrition, past obstetrical history and prenatal care.

Fifth or subsequent baby—after many births, the uterus and abdominal wall are more stretched, resulting in more malpresentations, cord prolapse and hemorrhage; polyhydramnios is also more common; tiredness and poor nutrition are often found as well.

Smoking—results in calcified spots on placenta, low birth weight babies, respiratory problems.

SELF-CHECK

1.   List the danger signs of pregnancy:
     a. _____
     _____
     b. _____
     _____
     c. _____
     _____
     d. _____
     _____
     e. _____
     _____

2.   If pregnant, with whom are you receiving prenatal care? Write down any questions you want to ask and haven't yet.

3.   What is protein in the urine a possible sign of?
     Glucose in the urine?
4.   What is edema?
5.   Are you Rh^+ or Rh^-?
6.   Why is it so important not to be anemic?
     How high should your hemoglobin count or hematocrit be for a home birth?
     What is your level?
     What foods are especially rich in iron (see next chapter)?
7.   What is the normal range of fetal heart tones?
     What is your baby's?
8.   If your baby is not head down by the eighth month, what exercise can you do?
9.   Do you have any medical factors that place you or your baby in the risk category? (describe)
     Have you discussed them with your birth attendant?
     Have you discussed them with your partner?
     Is there anything you can do to help the condition?
10. Write down any unresolved questions, feelings, doubts, options, etc. that you have:
     Discuss them with your partner.
     How can you get more information to help you in your decisions?

RECORD OF PRENATAL CARE

Name: _____   Birth Date: _____

Address: _____   Age: _____

Height: _____ Pre-pregnant weight: _____   Last menstrual period: _____

Estimated due date: _____   Was it normal: _____

Any bleeding since then: _____

Previous pregnancies: Number _____ Live births _____ Stillbirths _____

Miscarriages _____   Induced abortions _____

Date	Weeks Gest.	Wgt.	Urine: (protein, sugar, ketones)	Blood pressure	Height of fundus	Position of baby	Fetal heart tones	Edema	Other: fever, quickening, bleeding, headache, dizziness, nausea, tiredness, etc.	Next visit	Exam by

LABORATORY RESULTS

Test	Date	Results
VDRL (syphilis)		
Rh		
Rh antibody titer		
Rh antibody titer		
Blood type		
Hematocrit (hct) or Hemoglobin count		
Tine test		
Pap smear		
Vag strep		
Urinalysis		
Gonorrhea culture		
Rubella		
Other		

PELVIC ASSESSMENT:

Pubic arch _____

S/S notch _____

Coccyx _____

Largest baby delivered _____

Evaluation:

Conjugate/sacrum _____

Bi-ischial diameter _____

Ischial spines _____

PRENATAL HISTORY

YOUR MEDICAL HISTORY

Have you ever had (circle):
Rheumatic fever, heart trouble, dizziness or fainting, high blood pressure, anemia, epilepsy or convulsions, bladder infections, kidney infections, hepatitis, asthma, thyroid problems, German measles, diabetes, hypoglycemia, cancer, tuberculosis, "nervous breakdown," blood clotting problems, varicose veins, other:

Details: _____

_____

_____

Surgery: _____

Injuries: _____

Accidents: _____

Blood transfusions: _____

Are you currently taking any medications? _____

Do you use drugs? _____

Do you smoke? (amount): _____

Diet: _____ Vegetarian (type and how long): _____

_____ Non-vegetarian: _____

YOUR GYNECOLOGICAL HISTORY

Menstruation: Age began_____ No. days flow _____
No. days cycle _____
   Amount: light, medium, heavy. Regular or irregular?
   Have you ever had problems with (give dates and detail):

Painful cramping: _____

Excessive bleeding: _____

Venereal disease: _____

Gonorrhea: _____

Syphilis: _____

Other: _____

Herpes: _____

Vaginal infections: _____

Pelvic infections: _____

Difficulty in becoming pregnant: _____

Other (cysts, tumors, etc.): _____

Have you ever had a D&C? (dates and reason): _____
Have you ever had a suction abortion? _____

Most recent method of birth control: _____
    How long used? _____
    Side effects? _____
List any other methods of birth control you have used, how long, and any reactions to them: _____
_____

Previous Pregnancies:

    Number _____ Live births _____
    Stillbirths _____ Miscarriages _____
    Abortions _____

Problems during previous pregnancies:

	Number of pregnancy	Which trimester	Detail (including treatment)
Protein in urine			
Sugar in urine			
Anemia			
Spotting or bleeding			
Vaginal infections			
Edema (swelling)			
Morning sickness			
Continued nausea (2nd, 3rd trim.)			
Pre-eclampsia			
Eclampsia			
High blood pressure			
Bladder or kidney infection			
Varicose veins			
Prematurity			
Induced labor			
Episiotomy			
Tearing (stitches?)			
Difficulty with placenta			
Anesthesia			
Forceps			
Hemorrhage			
Depression after birth			
Problems with baby after birth			
Other			

Pregnancies ending in miscarriage or abortion:

Date	Miscarriage or Abortion	Length of Gestation	Difficulties

Previous Births:

No. _____ No. premature _____ No. now alive _____

Date	Sex	Birth weight	Home/ Hosp.	Length of labor	Medica- tions	Comments/ complications
1.						
2.						
3.						
4.						
5.						
6.						

FAMILY HISTORY

Has either your father, mother, siblings or other relatives ever had (circle):

High blood pressure, clots or bleeding, tuberculosis, kidney problems, congenital abnormalities, stroke, "heart trouble," diabetes (age discovered), cancer, twins (including father's family), other:

Details (who, outcome):

YOUR MOTHER'S
OBSTETRICAL HISTORY

How many children did your mother have? _____

How many born in hospital? _____

How many at home? _____

Were there any cesarean deliveries? _____

Breeches? _____

Any complications of pregnancy or birth? _____

What was her attitude toward birth? _____

Number of children she breastfed. _____

Any difficulties? _____

Did she take diethylstilbestrol while pregnant with you? Yes _____ No _____ Don't know _____

NOTES

SETH'S BIRTH

Rahima

Through the births of our two children and my constant involvement with birth, my own ideas have changed over the years. The story of Seth's birth, followed by Faith's later in the book, may give you some idea of that evolution.

I first became involved with childbirth in the spring of 1972. We had been on a spiritual search that had taken us as far as India. Sitting on a bus in Bombay just after leaving the ashram of a very holy man, I received the guidance that I was to be involved with birth and should write a book about the spiritual aspects of childbirth. At the time, I knew nothing about having a baby.

Several months later we began to investigate childbirth and felt that the time was right for us to open ourselves to conceiving. We were living at a Sufi center in the English countryside, and were fortunate to meet Sheila Kitzinger, who lived about ten miles away. I had read her book *The Experience of Childbirth* with great excitement and relief—so it really *was* possible to have a baby joyously instead of having to endure agony or be knocked out during childbirth.

When the time seemed right for us to have a baby, Wahhab and I did ablutions (ritual washing) asking for purification, and sat together in meditation, trying to open ourselves in service as instruments for the birth of a child, if it were God's will. During the first meditation, I had the intuition that we would have a boy and that his name would be Seth. I had no idea who Seth was, so afterwards I looked it up in the Bible and found that Seth, meaning *Gift of God*, was the third son of Adam, and the second patriarch. I was amazed a few months later to read in a class on Sufism that Seth was "the first manifestation of the Wahhab" (God's generosity).

We did ablutions and tried to be very clear every time we made love, and I felt as if I conceived that first month. When I had a light period two weeks later, I was tremendously disappointed, and even doubted my own spiritual insights. And then when I didn't conceive for six months, I went through a lot of changes. It was a time of purification and of burning my ego involvement with trying to have a baby, and with being a writer. For when we returned to the United States with the book synopsis, we discovered that the impulse towards a spiritual birth at home had not been a private one; several of the early books on homebirth had just come out, necessitating a complete revision of what we needed to include in "our book."

Once I gave up trying to become pregnant and left it in God's hands, I conceived immediately. Then, of course, my involvement with birth increased in fervor. I felt the burning question, "What is the best way for a child to be born so the spiritual qualities inherent in birth can manifest more fully?"

Several months later we were on a brief vacation in Paris. As we were about to return to London, our hostess said, "By the way, I don't know if you'd be interested, but I know an obstetrician who has developed a spiritual way of delivering babies." We abandoned our train tickets in order to be introduced to Dr. Frederick LeBoyer and learn of his deliveries without violence, which you can read about in Chapter 9.

I had always known I would have a homebirth; there was never any question in my mind. In England I encountered a little resistance about first babies, but I knew I would be able to find a good midwife. Everything seemed ideal.

However, when I was five months pregnant, we unexpectedly ended up settling in Los Angeles after two years abroad. In addition to other forms of culture shock, I had to figure out how I would have my baby at home in Los Angeles. After talking with everyone I met and spending several hours on the phone, I discovered that there were three chiropractors in Los Angeles doing homebirths, and we chose one of them. I was still of the opinion in those days that doctors delivered babies, so I never objected to the fact that he brought his own delivery table and sterile draping—at least it would be in our house. I was, however, upset even then by his great-white-father image. Every time I would ask questions or try to find out more about birth, he would say (with the best of intentions), "Don't be afraid, I'll take care of everything." I often cried on the way home from appointments because I felt so frustrated and misunderstood.

One of his standard procedures to which I did object was taking an x-ray with all first babies to see if the head would clear the pelvis. We kept wondering how we were going to get around it when Seth solved the problem for us; I went into labor the day it was supposed to be taken. I really felt that Seth didn't want to be subjected to it and decided to get out, ten days before my due date.

We hadn't found much active support for our decision to have a homebirth and went to a Lamaze class that consisted of nineteen hospital-bound couples and us. We and they were alternately appalled by each others' views, but we managed to get through the six weeks of classes. We remained amazed that no one objected to the descriptions of hospital procedures which came up in class. We were all learning to keep our eyes open and breathe during labor, but no one was really daring to be self-determined.

Labor began for me with surprising intensity. Returning from a Halloween party at midnight, I suddenly found myself with broken waters and contractions every five minutes. We phoned our doctor, who grudgingly drove the forty-five minutes to our home at 2 A.M. to find I was only 2 cm dilated. While he was scolding me for calling him out there, I hardly had a single contraction. I now know about psychological dystocia, in which feeling put down can slow or stop labor. But at the time I felt guilty, resentful and humiliated.

We took his advice, however, and went back to sleep for a few hours, until contractions again woke me around 6 A.M. and required Wahhab's active coaching. After a while I was having to do transition breathing and felt that I must be doing something wrong, because labor was painful and the doctor had said the baby wouldn't be born for hours and hours. Because I didn't look or feel like my image of the woman in the film I had seen on painless childbirth, I felt that I must have done something wrong, that I had somehow failed.

However, I actually *was* in transition, and when the doctor returned (without his nurse, because I certainly couldn't be that far along), he immediately set up his table for the delivery. What a relief it was to be pushing. I had a vague memory of Sheila Kitzinger writing that pushing need not be an athletic event, but I had been about to reread that section of her book when I went into labor ten days early. So I had to revert to the pushing we had practiced in Lamaze classes. Even though I panted for the crowning, I tore quite badly and was very sore through my shoulders the next day from pushing so hard.

Seth was born at 10:34 A.M. on November 1, 1973. The first words he heard were Wahhab whispering in his ear, "*La ilaha ill' Allah* (there is only One Being), but in the meantime your name is Seth Kenner Baldwin." The birth was an incredibly moving event. I never fully believed it was real or that I could have a baby until I held him in my arms. The images I had had of labor were of calmly lying naked next to Wahhab, sharing energy and enjoying the process together. However, by the time we were awake enough to be coherent, it was all we could do to keep everything together through transition, the more so since we didn't recognize it as transition (because I had been "hysterical" before and our doctor had said no delivery until late afternoon). We were thinking in desperation, "How are we ever going to get through seven more hours of this?" when we realized it was transition, our

friends arrived, our doctor arrived, and we were starting delivery all at the same instant. What a relief!

I had also had images of being surrounded by a group of friends for the birth. But when we left England and found ourselves in Los Angeles, we only invited our two closest friends to be with us. Even though part of me wanted a lot of people, and a photographer, another part of me lacked confidence and thought, "What if I make a fool of myself?" So we never even got a single photo of Seth's birth, which we regretted later.

I had no idea how I would experience giving birth, whether it would be ecstatic or religious or ordinary or what. Although I was unprepared for the intensity of transition, the birth itself was permeated by an incredible calm. In between pushing contractions and after Seth was born, the room was completely filled with a calmness I could almost see and touch.

Seth breathed right away, even before he was completely out. He let one cry out as he filled his lungs and then was totally calm and aware.

We had tried to explain to our doctor what we had learned from LeBoyer in Paris, even showing him LeBoyer's letters to us. Although he was basically open ("Once the baby is out, you can do whatever you want to do. I really go along with what couples want. If you want me to take off my shoes, or if you want to burn incense, that's fine with me.") We felt that he hadn't grasped the basic realization of what we were trying to do and why.

We didn't realize how incomplete our communication had been until the birth. Instead of a bulb syringe, he whipped out an electric suctioning device (for a baby who was already completely pink!). We were horrified: it hadn't even occurred to us to ask about *that*. I was pointing at my baby and vehemently whispering, "I want my baby!" (He had told us he always put the baby immediately up onto the mother's stomach . . .)

"Like that?" he asked. "You'll get all dirty!" We groaned inwardly and took Seth, caressing and massaging him. Wahhab cut the cord after it had stopped pulsing and did the LeBoyer bath with Seth.

Despite the few seconds delay due to the doctor's squeamishness, Seth was the first baby in the United States born with the direct use of LeBoyer's insights. The air of calm present at the birth stayed with Seth throughout most of his first year; he was amazingly happy and peaceful and almost never cried.

After I was stitched up, we were left alone with our new baby, which was wonderful, and with the realization of just having given birth and suddenly being parents, which was a real shock! My friend was unable to come the following week because she had just gotten a job; Wahhab had to go back to work the next day (we couldn't afford any deductions from his salary) so I was really left all alone, feeling that I ought to be able to handle everything and not really feeling up to it. I can't emphasize strongly enough the importance of having help and support during the first week.

We were really happy that Seth was born and that the birth had been at home and had gone so smoothly. But I was dissatisfied in several ways, realizing later that even though I had an awareness of the new being during my pregnancy, I had never really gained awareness of myself. Being the dogged and intrepid person that I am, however, I regrouped my self-image and vowed that before I had a second child I would get to the bottom of the "painless childbirth" mystery, understand why I tore, and have a community of support around me for the second birth. And so we did all that, although I never could have foreseen all of the changes I went through before Faith was born.

CHAPTER THREE

Nourishing Yourself and Your Baby: Nutrition and Exercise

ARE YOU WHAT YOU EAT?

Nutrition is an emotion-laden topic on which theories vary widely, as do individuals' eating habits. But no matter who your dietary guru is or what style of eating you're consciously or habitually following, there are certain areas of overwhelming consensus regarding the connection between diet and pregnancy.

Aside from the growth of very early childhood, pregnancy is the time of greatest change in your body. In addition, the patterns of growth set in your unborn baby's body at this time will affect his entire life.

By the time your first period is a couple of weeks late, your baby already has a rudimentary spinal cord and brain beginning to form and a heart that is beating on its own. In fact, the formation of most organs has begun, even though the embryo is only about a quarter of an inch long.

Since the construction of the baby's body and the changes in your own body all depend on food nutrients, the time of pregnancy is a time when you must be aware of what you are taking into your body even if normally you are completely oblivious to what you eat.

On the negative side, there is abundant evidence of the effects of poor nutrition on babies. They range from prematurity and low birth weight to brain damage and stillbirth. On the positive side, there is good evidence that healthy practices during pregnancy will lead to a stronger, healthier, more intelligent baby. So even though you probably won't change all your eating habits overnight, take advantage of the time of pregnancy to make a shift for the better on your "frontier area," whether by increasing the protein value of your diet, cutting down on sugars, or eating more fresh vegetables.

Among the areas of agreement of almost all schools of nutrition are the following:

1. Maternal nutrition has a profound effect on the developing fetus, on labor and delivery, and on postpartum recovery.

2. Pregnant and nursing mothers require a greater amount of every vitamin and mineral than before becoming pregnant.

3. There is a need for increased protein during pregnancy—between 75 and 100 grams per day. Protein is the building block of new tissue, which is both vital for your baby and is also necessary to prevent toxemia of pregnancy. Dr. Tom Brewer, whose work on toxemia we have already mentioned, has shown in over twenty-five years of working with toxemia that it is a disease resulting from metabolic disturbance, chiefly in the liver cells, and that it is caused by malnutrition, especially protein deficiency. Let me again recommend the book *What Every Pregnant Woman Should Know: The Truth about Diets and Drugs in Pregnancy* by Gail Sforza Brewer, which not only summarizes his work, but also includes menus and other recommendations for a healthy pregnancy and good prenatal care. If you're vegetarian, be sure to eat complete protein and be in touch with your body's increased need for protein even if you don't eat the above amount.

4. Everything you take in passes through the placenta and influences your baby either directly or indirectly. This means that caffeine, smoking and *all* drugs from aspirin to psychoactive drugs to obstetrical medication affect your unborn baby.

GETTING WHAT YOU NEED

Some schools of nutrition are opposed to the use of vitamin and mineral supplements, suggesting that you simply improve the quality of your diet so that it provides all your nutritional needs. Others, feeling that it is difficult by diet alone—especially considering vitamin losses caused by current methods of food growing, storage, transport and cooking—encourage the use of supplements. It's good to be sure, but we cannot depend on pills and powders to provide our nourishment. Body chemistry is immensely complex, and only very little understood. We do not know what essential vitamins and minerals are as yet undiscovered or what other subtle qualities exist in foods that come directly from living sources. And we do not know what complex interactions take place between our different foods.

Eating a wide variety of foods that grow naturally around us, chosen in consonance with what we know of their nutritional values, prepared in a way to maximize their flavor and minimize nutritional loss (e.g. by steaming rather than boiling), and complemented by food supplements if chosen, will give the best possible beginning to your baby's body.

NO, NOT THE FOUR BASIC FOOD GROUPS AGAIN

Like me, you have probably had the four basic food groups drilled into you from elementary school on, and as a result you now know that carrots are rich in vitamin A. I will not belabor these points. However, there are certain nutriments which are *crucial* during pregnancy. This section will discuss each of them in turn, giving a list of natural sources for them, a discussion of taking them as supplements, and a brief explanation of their importance.

IRON

Since it is hard to meet the extra demands your body has for iron from the third month of pregnancy on, iron supplements are usually recommended. In a normal pregnancy, you need 30 mg of iron daily. Of this, part goes to the developing fetus, and the rest goes to prevent anemia in your blood, which increases in volume by at least a quart during pregnancy. Iron tends to be constipating, but taking it with meals helps to counteract this. If your body is not absorbing the iron well, take smaller doses more frequently or try time-release iron. Taking 100 mg of vitamin C with each iron pill can also help it to be absorbed.

It is extremely important not to be anemic, because anemia compounds postpartum hemorrhage, can result in fetal distress in labor, and can cause weakness after the birth. You should have your blood checked at your first prenatal visit and again in the seventh or eighth month.

FOLIC ACID

Liver and other organ meats, nuts, nutritional (torula) yeast, leafy green vegetables, oysters, salmon, whole grains, mushrooms.

Folic acid is one of the B vitamins. Your body requires double its normal amount during pregnancy, so you should check that any prenatal vitamins you are taking contain it. Its deficiency is associated with hemorrhage and premature separation of the placenta.

VITAMIN B^{12}

Cheese, milk, milk products, fish, organ meats, eggs. This will only be lacking if a person has been a complete vegetarian for years. It is important because its lack causes anemia. Vegetarians can take yeast which has been especially prepared to contain B^{12} or separate vitamin B^{12} tablets. Tempeh, a soy product, contains B^{12}.

CALCIUM

Dairy products, almonds, cracked sesame seeds or tahini, canned fish with bones, soybeans or tofu. Buy a supplement with half as much magnesium as calcium. You need 1200 mg/day of calcium.

PROTEIN

Meats, poultry, fish, whole grains, legumes (peas, beans, lentils, etc.), nuts, seeds, dairy products (milk, yoghurt, cheese, cottage cheese), eggs. Because protein is so important, let us explore it in greater detail.

INCREASING THE PROTEIN VALUE OF WHAT YOU EAT

Your need for protein approximately doubles while you are pregnant, between 75 and 100 grams per day. Protein is vital in the formation of your baby's body and in preventing toxemia in pregnancy.

Certainly you don't think you're malnourished. But what do you really eat? Think about what you've actually eaten in the last twenty-four hours. Was each meal nutritionally sound, or was there an exception, like skimping on a meal because you were late in the morning or were downtown at lunch time? The statement, "This day isn't typical because. . ." probably indicates more exceptions than are good for the two of you. To get a picture of your eating habits, fill in the worksheets at the end of this section, (see p. 41) and then act on the results you see!

Vegetarians especially need to be sure they are receiving adequate protein from their diet, with added iron and calcium and a good prenatal vitamin/mineral supplement. Grain protein alone is not sufficient—your diet needs to include high quality protein such as soy or dairy products. Complete vegetarians will need to supplement vitamin B^{12}, as mentioned.

Proteins are classified as either complete or incomplete, according to the number and ratio of essential amino acids present. Complete proteins contain all eight essential amino acids in a balance close to the proportion in which our body requires them. Animal protein (meat, milk and cheese, eggs) and soybeans rank high in net protein utilization. Other vegetable proteins (peas, beans, lentils, nuts, etc.) are fairly incomplete sources of protein, but the amount of usable protein they provide can be greatly increased by eating foods from the two groups at the same time or by combining complementary vegetable proteins at the same meal.

EXAMPLES OF COMPLEMENTARY PROTEIN COMBINATIONS

Wheat and milk	Soybeans and millet
Rice and milk	Peanuts and sunflower seeds
Rice and legumes	Beans and corn
Wheat and legumes	Beans and milk
Rice and sesame seeds	Peanuts and milk

The book *Diet for a Small Planet* by Frances Moore Lappe discusses complementary proteins and fulfilling protein requirements from a vegetarian perspective, while the companion book, *Recipes for a Small Planet* by Ellen Buchman Ewald, gives recipes and menus which implement those ideas.

DISCOVERING SOY PRODUCTS: FOR VEGETARIANS AND NON-VEGETARIANS

Soybeans and soy products are very high in protein, containing all eight essential amino acids. Soy is economical, versatile and delicious.

Although you may not have liked soybeans by themselves, they can be made into soyburgers or loaves and are delicious served with various sauces. And the exciting thing is that soy can be transformed in a great many ways, including tofu and miso (two essential ingredients of the oriental diet), soy flour, grits, soy milk, yoghurt, cheese, sprouts, etc. I recommend *The Book of Tofu* by Shurtleff and Aoyagi, an enjoyable and informative book with every imaginable use for tofu (all of them delicious), and *The Farm Vegetarian Cookbook* for a delicious introduction to the versatility of soy.

Tempeh, a fermented soybean patty with a nutty flavor, is even richer in protein than tofu and has high levels of vitamin B_{12}.

SOME THINGS TO AVOID

Alcohol Alcohol quickly crosses the placenta, and definitely affects the baby. Although up to two drinks in a day may not have any lasting effect on either your baby or you, heavy drinking can cause the baby to develop a series of birth defects known as *fetal alcohol syndrome.*

Smoking Babies of smokers tend to be smaller and have more respiratory problems and other difficulties in the first year. Smokers also have higher miscarriage rates in the first trimester and a higher stillborn rate. Smoking is especially harmful during the second half of pregnancy, stunting the baby's growth either by restricting placental circulation or by the direct effect of nicotine on the baby.

Any Kind of Drug All drugs affect your baby. Medications should be under a physician's and *your* strict supervision. Antibiotics cross the placenta quickly; tetracycline may cause discoloration of your baby's permanent teeth and may affect bone growth; some sulfa drugs can disturb the baby's liver function. If you have a stubborn infection, let a doctor *who knows you are pregnant* prescribe, or see a naturopath or herbalogist. Daily aspirin use also results in a higher rate of complications in labor and delivery, including hemorrhage and infection and anemia during pregnancy.

Excessive Caffeine Studies have shown that caffeine causes birth defects when animals are exposed to moderately high levels, levels to which some pregnant women might expose themselves. More research is needed on the possible role of caffeine in human birth defects, miscarriages and infertility. Caffeine is found in coffee, black and green tea, mate, and cola drinks.

Foods with artificial colors, flavors, additives, preservatives, or artificial sweeteners; also nitrates and nitrites as in hot dogs, luncheon meats and bologna.

You'll do your baby and your body a favor by avoiding these.

Foods high in calories and low in food value.

SOME PROBLEMS OF PREGNANCY AFFECTED BY DIET

TOXEMIA

Many doctors have prescribed low-calorie, low-salt diets in an attempt to limit weight gain and swelling, thought to be early signs of toxemia. This is the wrong treatment, asserts Dr. Brewer, and in the chapter "Understanding Swelling: Water Retention is Normal;" the Brewers relate that 80 to 90 percent of women swell up at some time in the course of their pregnancies.[1]

This physiological swelling is not a sign of toxemia per se, and salt restriction and diuretics are not indicated according to Dr. Brewer's research and other testimony before the FDA hearing on diuretics.

If you are having marked swelling, check with your doctor, check your diet, and read the Brewers' book (they recommend you keep salting foods to taste, as normal salt intake is needed to maintain the increased blood volume of pregnancy required for sufficient placental circulation).

WEIGHT GAIN

A generation ago, weight gain was strictly limited by doctors to 8–10 pounds. It was later discovered that babies (and mothers) were being undernourished. Then the magic number became 24 pounds, or about a half a pound a week.

This is no longer true. A gain of 35 pounds (or more with twins) on a high-protein diet is healthy.

When I was pregnant with Seth, my homebirth doctor still wielded the tyranny of the scales, and I gained exactly twenty-four pounds. It was a surprisingly uplifting experience to be pregnant with Faith in Mexico and have the midwife say, "You're so big. You're huge! It's wonderful that you're so big and healthy."

You do need to watch what you're eating—that it's well balanced, high in protein, and doesn't contain foods that add calories and little or no food value. But you don't need to gain a strict half-pound a week.

NAUSEA OR MORNING SICKNESS

If morning sickness plagues you in the first few months of pregnancy, try eating some kind of carbohydrate,

like whole wheat toast, before getting up in the morning. Drink lots of water to avoid dehydration, and try to eat smaller amounts more frequently (even every two hours until your system settles again). Taking 100 mg of vitamin B[6] daily often helps, as does not dwelling on your condition (it almost always disappears by the end of the third month). Ginger has also been helpful.

INDIGESTION

As your baby grows, your stomach and intestines are being squeezed into ever smaller spaces, and the progesterone in your system also causes the muscles of your stomach to relax, so that heartburn is not uncommon. Try to avoid extremely spicy foods, and eat smaller amounts more often. Alfalfa tablets or alfalfa tea often help, and peppermint tea is also good for digestion.

CONSTIPATION AND HEMORRHOIDS

Constipation is common in pregnancy, due to the relaxing effect of progesterone on the entire gastrointestinal tract. Iron supplements often add to the problem. The condition can be helped by drinking more liquids (eight or more glasses a day, including milk, water, juices, soups, etc.), and eating foods high in bulk, such as wheat bran, whole grain breads and cereals, dried and fresh fruits, raw vegetables, and salads. Prune juice helps; anything stronger should be taken only on advice from your doctor and shouldn't be necessary if you work on diet first.

To prevent straining and hemorrhoids, keep a small stepstool or box by the toilet to put your feet on so your knees are higher than your hips. Then when having a bowel movement, *release* the pelvic floor, sit up straight, and block with the diaphragm by holding your breath. It's much better for you and is good practice for the way you will push in labor. If hemorrhoids are troublesome, you can use an astringent such as witch hazel, alum or "Tucks" pads. Hemorrhoid cream or suppositories without hydrocortisone can be used.

LEG CRAMPS

Cramps in the calves are caused by poor circulation and buildup of lactic acid. If you get a cramp, flex your toe up toward your chin and rub the calf. Increasing your calcium supplement or taking vitamin E sometimes helps prevent cramps.

OTHER CHANGES DURING PREGNANCY

FREQUENT URINATION

In early pregnancy you may think, "My baby's only an inch long and already I'm peeing every few hours!"

---

[1]Gail Sforza Brewer with Tom Brewer, M.D. *What Every Pregnant Woman Should Know: The Truth About Diets and Drugs in Pregnancy* (New York: Random House, 1977), pp. 34–41)

What happens is that the expanding uterus falls forward onto the bladder, and the relaxant effects of progesterone also signal frequent urination. Getting up at night is good preparation for getting up later with the baby!

VARICOSE VEINS

Varicose veins are increased during pregnancy due to the effects of progesterone on the blood vessels and due to the pressing of the uterus against the main blood vessels returning from the legs.

Standing a great deal is not good for your circulation, but walking is. Lying with your legs up on pillows two or three times a day and putting blocks under the foot of your bed can help. Sitting with your legs up and avoiding hard wooden chairs also helps. Don't sit with your legs crossed at the knee, which impairs circulation. Tailor-sitting on the floor with your legs crossed is ideal, not only for circulation, but also for helping prepare your muscles for birth (squatting also helps tone your pelvic floor muscles).

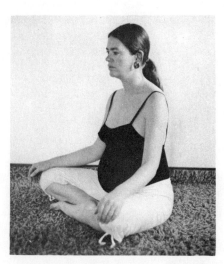

FIGURE 3-1. *Sitting cross-legged helps your circulation.*

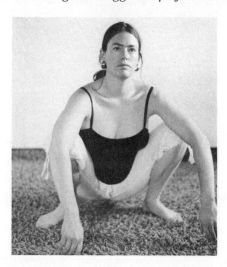

FIGURE 3-2. *Squatting helps your pelvic floor muscles.*

If you do need support stockings during pregnancy, put them on before putting your legs over the side of the bed in the morning, before blood has flowed down into them.

Some sources state that vitamin E helps varicose veins. Recommended dosage is two 400-IU capsules a day for two weeks, then one 400-IU capsule daily.

TIREDNESS

Tiredness often occurs in the first few months and then improves in the second trimester. Nap in the afternoon, and get sufficient rest at night. Your body is going through a lot more changes than are apparent externally.

STRETCH MARKS

They aren't so likely if you eat well and don't gain an excessive amount of weight. Using a cream or natural oil and massaging your stomach is good for the skin and also puts you more in touch with your baby. Vitamin E cream is especially recommended.

Some women develop a *linea negra* or dark line of pigmentation down from the belly button; other women have darker pigmentation on their face during pregnancy (the so-called mask of pregnancy).

CHANGES IN THE BREASTS

Tenderness of the breasts and a darkening of the areola accompany pregnancy. Your breasts develop and increase in size as your baby develops, and hormones cause the tissues to stretch, so you may find a bra more comfortable in later pregnancy even if you haven't worn one in years. If you buy a nursing bra late in pregnancy, you can use it when your milk comes in—when you'll definitely need the support.

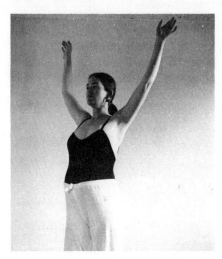

FIGURE 3-3. *Arm circles exercise.*

In order to help strengthen the pectoral muscles, which support the breasts, you can do arm circles, also known as the lactation exercise.

Arm Circles

Stand with feet parallel, shoulder width apart, arms straight out to the sides, palms facing forward. Take a deep cleansing breath, hold, and exhale. Make five large circles, inhaling with each circle. Now circle the opposite direction five times, exhaling with each circle. Repeat. This exercise strengthens your shoulder and upper back muscles as well as toning the pectoral muscles. It also helps ventilate the lungs and can help with shortness of breath.

PRE-LABOR CONTRACTIONS

Your uterus is contracting all the time, but you usually only feel it in the last month or so (or earlier if this is not your first baby). Occasionally the contractions are strong enough to seem like labor, but they don't dilate the cervix and will usually stop if you change your position or type of activity.

VAGINAL DISCHARGE

Mucous discharge usually increases with pregnancy. Wearing cotton underwear (or none at all) will help let air in. If discharge becomes more profuse and itches, you may have a yeast infection (pregnancy changes your vaginal environment so yeast are more likely to grow in it). Acidophilus capsules in the vagina can help; avoid iodine douches.

DIZZINESS

Hormones cause your blood vessels to relax, making it more difficult to get blood up to your brain. And the velocity of your venous blood flow in your legs is decreased by two-thirds when you are sitting, so always get up slowly rather than springing up. And as you become more pregnant, always roll to the side and use your hands when lying down and getting up rather than straining your abdominal muscles.

Egg Roll

When lying down, "walk down" on your hands, then roll onto your back. To get up, roll onto your side and "walk up."

EMOTIONS

You may find early in pregnancy that your emotions are much closer to the surface or that your head seems a

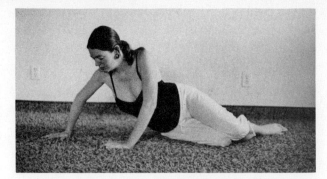

FIGURE 3-4. *Egg roll exercise.*

little fuzzy. You may feel introverted, irritable or unusually weepy. The emotional roller-coastering of pregnancy is related to hormonal changes your body is going through; but don't get self-indulgent. Pregnancy is an ideal time for growth. The exercises in *Pregnant Feelings* by Baldwin and Palmarini can be very helpful.

BACKACHE

Lower backache is a common complaint of pregnancy as the growing uterus pulls more and more on the broad ligaments connecting it to the sacrum. Stand straight, with your buttocks slightly tucked to counteract the tendency to curve the back forward.

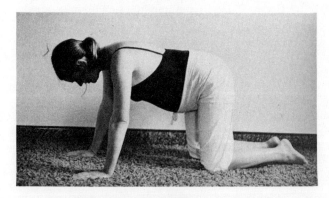

FIGURE 3-5. *Pelvic rock (a).*

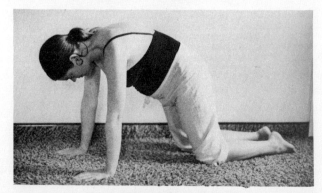

FIGURE 3-6. *Pelvic rock (b).*

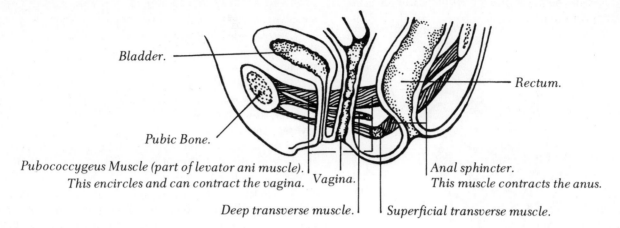

Bladder.

Rectum.

Pubic Bone.

Pubococcygeus Muscle (part of levator ani muscle).
This encircles and can contract the vagina.   Vagina.

Anal sphincter.
This muscle contracts the anus.

Deep transverse muscle.

Superficial transverse muscle.

FIGURE 3-7.

Pelvic Rocks

This exercise can really help alleviate lower back pain. Get on your hands and knees with your back at right angles, like a table. Rock your pelvis by tucking your buttocks under. This will round your lower back. Release. Repeat about twenty times. All of the movement is in the pelvis, not in the shoulders or upper back.

EXERCISE DURING PREGNANCY

Not only does sufficient exercise during pregnancy help you feel your best, but your baby also appreciates the increased circulation and oxygenation. Outdoor work and activity are excellent, but many people don't have a lifestyle which provides them with adequate physical activity.

If you find you don't get enough activity, yoga (avoiding upside-down postures), dance, Tai Chi Ch'uan, or other forms of non-violent whole body movement which also open up the breath are highly recommended. In many areas prenatal exercise classes are offered, and there are several good books listed at the end of this chapter. Such classes are excellent not only to orient you to your changing body and help prepare you for giving birth, but also for the emotional interchange they provide with other pregnant women. If none are available in your area, why not get a group of pregnant women together to form a pregnancy support group and see what backgrounds and resources you have among yourselves in terms of movement, massage, and so forth.

If you are used to some sport or other form of activity, by all means continue it while you are pregnant. Swimming is a favorite because it completely supports your body, lets you expend a lot of energy, and helps you feel refreshed and graceful. Activities such as horseback riding or bicycling should be discontinued once your center of gravity has shifted enough to make falls more likely. With anything you undertake let your body be your guide, and don't do anything that hurts, strains, or feels unsafe to you.

PELVIC FLOOR EXERCISES

The trampoline-like muscles of the pelvic floor cross the bottom of your pelvis and support your internal organs. These muscles are in several layers (Figure 3-7). The tone of these muscles is important to prevent urine from leaking out (if you urinate a little when you sneeze or cough, your pelvic floor is in disastrous condition!), to prevent constipation, and to keep the uterus from prolapsing, or sliding down (or even out of) the vagina. These conditions are not uncommon in older women who have had many children and who don't know about the pelvic floor exercises to restore tone to their muscles.

It is especially important that these muscles are in good tone for pregnancy and birth, because they not only need to support the weight of the expanding uterus, but they also need to stretch around the baby's head without tearing during birth.

The most important of these muscles is the pubococcygeal muscle, which has three parts: one going from the pubic bone in a horseshoe loop around the back of the vagina; the other going into and around the back of the rectum; and the third attaching to the tailbone (Figure 3-8).

There are simple exercises you can do to assure that the PCG muscle is in good condition for the birth and will tighten up again after your baby is born. You can learn what contracting this muscle feels like by trying to squeeze your partner's penis during intercourse. You may find that when you try contracting and holding the

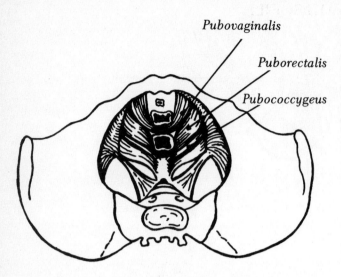

Pubovaginalis

Puborectalis

Pubococcygeus

FIGURE 3-8.

muscle now you also feel sexual sensation. One of the accompanying discoveries of Dr. Arnold Kegel's work with this muscle in cases of urinary incontinence was an increase in the frequency of women's orgasms. Because there are sexual receptors in this muscle surrounding the vagina, having it in tone can change your entire sexual experience.

You can also learn to isolate this muscle by trying to stop the flow of urine while sitting on the toilet, without contracting your legs or any other external muscles. Your pelvic floor has several layers of muscles which you can contract, including one at the opening of the vagina. The PCG muscle, however, is further up the vagina and is quite strong. You can try squeezing your

own finger and feeling the pressure of this muscle, but squeezing your partner is more fun.

Exercise 1. Sitting where you are, imagine the pelvic floor is like an elevator, and *slowly* bring it up to the second floor. Then slowly keep contracting up to the third, and then the fourth floor and hold, with the "elevator" all the way up to the top. Now slowly release and go back down through each floor. Release, and repeat several times each day.

Exercise 2. Contract your PCG muscle to a count of six, hold for four, and then release gradually. In order to get your pelvic floor in shape, you should do this exercise 200 times a day for six weeks, and then whenever you think of it during the rest of your pregnancy. After your baby is born, do it intensively again during the first six weeks, and then some every day for the rest of your life.

How can you do 200 a day? Easy, if you do them in groups of ten and set yourself certain reminders to do ten every time the phone rings, every time you stop at a red light, or every time you open the refrigerator. After the birth, you can do ten exercises every time you sit down to nurse or change the baby's diaper.

Exercise 3. Do the elevator exercise again, except this time as you come down to the ground floor, extend the muscles down into the "basement." Then come back up to the first floor, and release (always leave the muscle with good tone). This exercise can give you a preview of pushing your baby out, which involves releasing and extending the muscles of the pelvic floor.

For further discussion and exercises involving the pelvic floor, see *The Experience of Childbirth* by Sheila Kitzinger (New York: Penguin, 5th ed., 1984, pp. 48–51 and 155–158).

NUTRITIONAL PROFILE

Fill out the following form to gain a picture of your own eating habits; show it to your birth attendant for further counselling.

	Almost every day	3–4 times a week	Once or twice a week	Almost never
I usually eat:				
Breakfast				
Canned vegetables				
Frozen vegetables				
Fresh vegetables				
Leafy green				
Yellow or orange				
Fresh fruit				
Cheese				
Eggs				
Red meat				
Liver				
Fish				
Chicken				
Cooked soybeans				
Tofu				
Nuts, peanut butter, tahini, etc.				
Other sources of protein?				
Whole grains, whole wheat noodles, corn tortillas				
White rice, spaghetti, noodles				
Items with refined sugar (candy, cake, cookies, etc.)				
Carbonated beverages				

In a typical day, I eat:

_____ pieces of white bread

_____ pieces of whole grain bread

_____ glasses of milk (include milk in cooking, on cereal, yoghurt, etc.)

_____ at least one of the following (circle):
   orange, orange juice, cantaloupe, tomato, sprouts

_____ cups of (circle):
   coffee, black tea, herbal tea,
other _____

I am taking the following nutritional supplements:

_____ prenatal vitamins (do they include folic acid? _____)

_____ iron (type and dosage:_____)

_____ calcium (amount: _____)

_____ protein (amount and brand: _____)

_____ nutritional yeast (with vitamin B^{12} if complete vegetarian? _____)

Other foods that I usually like to eat during the week that are not already included are: _____
_____

I smoke about
_____ cigarettes a day.

NUTRITIONAL PROFILE: PROTEIN

Write down everything that you have eaten for the last three meals, including snacks. When you are finished, do the same for yesterday. Tomorrow, again record everything (or if you forget tomorrow, do it the next time you pick up the book).

	TODAY	YESTERDAY	THIRD DAY
Snack			
Breakfast			
Snack			
Lunch			
Snack			
Dinner			
Snack			

Now look up the protein values of the foods in the tables which follow, and write them next to the item. What are your protein totals?

Day 1: _____ grams
Day 2: _____ grams
Day 3: _____ grams

How can you improve the amount of protein you eat? Pregnant women need 75–100 grams of protein every day.

PROTEIN VALUES OF COMMON FOODS

The following list can give you a rough idea whether you are even approaching the 75–100 grams of protein a day which pregnant women need. For a more detailed table, see *What Every Pregnant Woman Should Know*, (Brewer, Random House, 1977) from which these values were taken.

	Serving size	Grams protein
Dairy Products		
Butter	1 pat	0
Hard cheeses	1 oz.	6–7
Cottage cheese	½ c.	15
Ricotta cheese	½ c.	19
Cream cheese	1 oz.	2
Egg	1	6
Milk (whole or skim)	1 c.	8–9
Yoghurt	1 c.	8

Meat and Poultry (serving is for cooked, edible portion without bones)

Beef		
Chuck roast	4 oz.	23
Corned beef	4 oz.	22
Dried, chipped	4 oz.	25
Ground, lean	4 oz.	22
Sirloin steak	4 oz.	20
Bologna	2 slices	7
Chicken or turkey	4 oz.	23
Duck	4 oz.	13
Lamb	4 oz.	18–20
Liver (beef or chicken)	4 oz.	20
Pork		
Bacon, crisp	1 slice	2
Pork chop	4 oz.	16
Ham slice, cured	4 oz.	16
Hotdog	1	7
Loin, roast	4 oz.	21
Sausage	4 oz.	11
Veal	4 oz.	23

Seafood (cooked, edible portion)

Fillet of white fish (baked or fried)	4 oz.	20–25
Crabmeat, cooked	4 oz.	14
Salmon	4 oz.	24–25
Sardines, canned	1 oz.	5
Shrimp, cleaned, steamed	4 oz.	20
Tuna, canned	4 oz.	28

Nuts and Seeds

Almonds	1 c.	21
Cashews	1 c.	19
Peanuts, roasted	1 c.	30
Peanut butter	⅓ c.	13
Pinenuts	1 c.	35
Sesame seeds	⅓ c.	5
Sunflower seeds (hulled)	½ c.	13
Walnuts	1 c.	17

Dried beans

Black-eyed peas (cowpeas)	4 oz. dry	25
Chick-peas (garbanzos)	1 c. cooked	16
Kidney beans	1 c. cooked	11
Lentils	⅓ c. dry	17
Navy or pinto beans	1 c. cooked	17
Split peas	1 c. cooked	11
Soybeans	1 c. cooked	26
Soybean curd (tofu)	4. oz.	9
Soybean sprouts	4 oz.	7

Flours and Grains (figures are for uncooked amounts)

Barley	½ c.	10
Cornflakes	⅔ c.	2
Corn grits or cornmeal	½ c.	10–11
Oats, rolled	¼ c.	4
Popcorn, popped	2 c.	3
Rice, brown	⅓ c.	5
Soy flour (full fat)	1 c.	41
Whole wheat flour	1 c.	15
Wheatena	¼ c.	4

Pasta (uncooked)

Egg noodles	1 c.	7
Macaroni or spaghetti (Buitoni high protein)	2 oz.	12

Fruit (All fruit servings have 2 gm, 1 gm or only trace protein except for the following:)

Dried apricots	4 oz.	5
Avocado	1 lg.	4
Dates, dried & pitted	1 c.	4
Figs, dried	3 lg.	3
Stewed prunes	1 c.	3

Vegetables (Vegetable servings with more than 2 gm protein include:)

Lima beans	1 c.	8
Broccoli, cooked	1 c.	5
Brussels sprouts, cooked	1 c.	6
Cauliflower, cooked	1 c.	3
Collard or dandelion greens	1 c. cooked	5
Corn on cob	1 ear	3
cooked loose	1 c.	5
Kale, cooked	1 c.	4

Mustard and turnip greens	1 c. cooked	3–4
Peas, fresh or frozen	1 c.	5
canned	1 c.	3
Potato		
boiled or baked	1 med.	2
hash browns	¾ c.	4
chips or French fries	10	1
Spinach, cooked	1 c.	3
Squash, winter cooked	1 c.	4
Squash, summer cooked	1 c.	1

Beverages
Non-milk beverages essentialy have little or no protein; exceptions:

Bouillon (canned)	1 c.	5
Orange and tomato juice	1 c.	2

Sweeteners

Honey, sugar, molasses, etc.		0

FOR FURTHER READING

PREGNANCY AND PRENATAL CARE

Heart and Hands: A Midwife's Guide by Elizabeth Davis. Very detailed and readable guide to prenatal care and birth.

The Complete Book of Pregnancy and Childbirth by Sheila Kitzinger. A comprehensive book by one of our favorite childbirth educators, developer of the psycho-sexual approach to childbirth education.

Pregnant Feelings by Rahima Baldwin and Terra Palmarini. Self-help guide to exploring issues and emotions of pregnancy to make it a time of inner transformation.

Prenatal Tests by Robin Blatt. A guide to their benefits and risks and how to decide whether or not to have them.

Spiritual Midwifery by Ina May Gaskin has two excellent sections on prenatal care and preparation, one for parents and one from the point of view of the birth attendant.

The Tentative Pregnancy by Barbara Katz Rothman. An exploration of prenatal tests and their psychological effects on women.

What Every Pregnant Woman Should Know: The Truth about Diet and Drugs in Pregnancy by Gail Sforza Brewer. Revised edition of this important book detailing Dr. Tom Brewer's work on toxemia and the recommendations for prevention.

PRENATAL EXERCISE

Essential Exercises for the Childbearing Year by Elizabeth Noble. One of the most thorough explorations of the physiology of pregnancy and movement, from pregnancy through postpartum.

Positive Pregnancy Through Yoga by Sylvia Klein Olkin. Olkin has developed Positive Pregnancy Fitness workshops, tapes and other resources.

Pregnant? *Bodywork I* is an excellent video with gentle detail pelvic floor, abdominal and back work. From Winter Green, P.O. Box 11830, Reno, NV 89510.

Prepare and Celebrate. Pre- and Post-natal exercise video. From Katherine DaSilva Jain. 5 Mt. Tioga Court, San Raphael, CA 94903.

NUTRITION

See bibliography at end of book.

CHAPTER FOUR

Planning for the Birth

YOUR BIRTH ATTENDANT

THE IMPORTANCE OF A SKILLED BIRTH ATTENDANT

Although 95 percent of low-risk births proceed completely normally without intervention, for the other 5 percent a skilled birth attendant is invaluable. She can help recognize the early signs of danger, offer advice about going to the hospital, and help with an emergency in the small percentage of cases when one arises. For even though prepared couples understand more about birth than couples previously have, it is still difficult, without extensive theoretical and practical skills and experience, to tell which situations are within the broad range of "normal" and which require medical attention.

Thus in a normal birth an attendant can help keep a homebirth at home through reassurance that everything is all right and by handling some situations which require attention without the need to go to a hospital. She can also help with coaching, especially when the father needs to eat or rest. And she can share her skills and compassion gained from attending many births and having had children herself (if your attendant is a man, it is still beneficial to have such a woman present as trusted friend, labor coach, etc.).

And having a skilled attendant can be especially important if something does go wrong; you have another opinion based on greater experience with birth and you can often save valuable time by early detection and action. In the event of a real emergency, your birth attendant should be skilled in emergency first-aid measures and may bring emergency equipment. In such a situation, having someone present who is skilled and experienced in birth and at the same time attuned with the current situation can be an invaluable and life-sav-

ing combination. I strongly urge that you find and use a skilled birth attendant, without giving up your responsibility to her, to help reduce the risks of homebirth to the inevitable minimum of nature.

DIFFERENT KINDS OF ATTENDANTS

Depending on where you live, you may have many kinds of birth attendants to choose from. If there is a doctor in your area who has a homebirth practice, make an appointment to talk with him, find out who he is and what his practice involves. The advantages of a doctor are continuity of care (in case of emergency he should have hospital privileges), greater familiarity with emergency equipment and procedures, and the ability to handle certain complications at home (suturing, etc). The disadvantages can be less familiarity with normal birth and more tendency to intervene or to want standard procedures such as prepping, enema, etc. And few doctors are willing to become involved in your labor as a midwife does.

In some states chiropractors are licensed to do deliveries, and osteopaths are able to do births in many states and may be more open to homebirth than M.D.s.

Many states license certified nurse-midwives to do deliveries as part of an obstetrical team. You may find them doing homebirths under a doctor's auspices or working in a birth center. Midwives have the orientation of helping a woman throughout pregnancy, labor and delivery, and if they are doing homebirths they probably haven't lost their orientation to normal birth during their training. They are able to administer drugs for hemorrhage; they can do episiotomies, suturing, etc., and they are trained in other emergencies, such as infant resuscitation. Because they are usually doing homebirths under a doctor's guidance, they have emergency backup and could remain with you in the hospital should any complications arise.

Lay or empirical midwives are women who are skilled in birth without first becoming a nurse. Although training programs are beginning to develop in several states, most empirical midwives have gained their training through self-study, apprenticing with another midwife, and through experience (hence the designation *empirical*). Laws in individual states may determine whether a lay midwife is able to practice openly, has doctor backup, carries emergency equipment, charges for her services, etc. Advantages tend to be an orientation toward normal birth, involvement in the entire labor and delivery, respect for the parents' decisions and experience; disadvantages can be lack of experience with complications, lack of good backup, and needing to go to the hospital for situations such as suturing.

Laws governing the practice of empirical and nurse midwives vary from state to state and are changing rapidly as more and more states legalize and regulate midwifery. To find out the current laws in your state, you can contact your local health department, purchase a booklet from Mothering Publications, Box 1690, Santa Fe, NM 87504, or write to the Midwives Alliance of North America, P.O. Box 175, Newton, KS 67114

If no one is openly doing homebirths in your area, you will have to do some searching to find your birth attendant. But with a bit of effort, it's surprising what resources you can discover.

How to Find a Skilled Attendant

Your first lead might be to talk with childbirth educators and La Leche League leaders and ask who is doing homebirths, which doctors are sympathetic for prenatal care, and so forth. (La Leche League has the official policy of never endorsing or recommending anything, but leaders tend to know everything that's happening in a community). Get their numbers from doctor's offices, hospitals, or the Red Cross.

In my opinion, it is good to talk to doctors about homebirth—it lets them know what consumers want. But remember that you are doing it as a service to them and don't be discouraged by the lectures you may receive. And who knows, you may be the one to radicalize a doctor, especially if he comes to know you through prenatal care first.

Next, talk to everyone you meet who looks like they might be involved with homebirth. Maybe they'll know someone. You can write up index cards stating something like, "I'm having my baby at home and would appreciate information from women who have had homebirths, or from anyone who has experience with births." Put these up in health food stores, free clinics, bookstores or wherever there are appropriate bulletin boards.

You may feel as if you're the only person in your area who cares about homebirth, but it isn't true. I am convinced that if you have strong intention and put out the energy, you will be given exactly the help you need. For example, when I first came to Boulder, Colorado, no one knew of anyone except one osteopath who was openly doing home deliveries. Within a few months of teaching classes, I had discovered two foreign-trained midwives who had each delivered 5,000 babies, and other people who would help at home deliveries including three obstetrical nurses, two physician's assistants, three lay midwives, and one M.D. who would occasionally do homebirths.

What if you don't find any help? You might be satisfied with delivering at a birth center or doing a hospital delivery with a sympathetic doctor and then going home a few hours after the birth (signing yourself out "against medical advice" if necessary). Athough I can't recommend homebirth without a skilled attendant, I recognize that some couples will be determined to do it even though they haven't found help. (Most unattended homebirths are not due to the couple's negligence, but result from the fact that doctors and legislators in many states refuse to recognize the rights of couples to give birth in their own homes with competent medical aid and emergency backup.) My advice in this case is that you *please* don't attempt it with just the two of you. There's too much to know and do, even in a normal birth, for the husband to be able to handle everything comfortably. And if complications occur, you can be in real trouble. At the very least involve friends, including women who have given birth, so that there will be help with coaching, cooking, looking after children, and so there will be help in an emergency situation (like taking the mother to the hospital in the knee-chest position, watching the baby if the mother has third-stage complications, etc.). And as a group, meet together often, study and prepare yourselves as much as possible. Be as responsible as you can, and don't stop looking for the help and information you need!

Skills of a Birth Attendant

With diligence and clear intention, most couples are able to find several sources of possible help. Having an experienced birth attendant is important, but it's equally important that you have a realistic appraisal of your attendant's skills and orientation toward birth. Our cultural conditioning is to accept unthinkingly the superiority of the expert and to discount our own knowledge and intuition. Doing this at a birth, whether the "expert" is an obstetrician or your next-door neighbor, will very likely lead to disappointment or disaster.

At a minimum, your birth attendant should be able to:

1. Recognize which prenatal factors place a woman or baby at risk and may contra-indicate a home delivery.

2. Know how to monitor labor, including checking dilation, the position of the baby, fetal heart tones and maternal blood pressure.

3. Recognize variations from a normal labor and know whether they can be managed at home or require hospitalization. (She also needs to participate in formulating your emergency backup plan.)

4. Know how to help the head to be born without tearing the perineum or vagina. She should know how to recognize degrees of tearing, should they occur, and be able to get them handled.

5. Check the placenta, umbilical cord and membranes.

6. Check the uterus for contraction after the birth and be able to recognize and handle hemorrhage.

7. Know how to check the newborn and recognize health problems.

8. Know how to handle critical emergencies such as shock, hemorrhage, shoulder dystocia, and how to give cardio-pulmonary resuscitation to the baby.

Ideally, there should be an almost telepathic sense of unity with your birth attendant. After all, you are going to be sharing one of the most intimate experiences of your life with this person.

SELECTING A SKILLED ATTENDANT

Once you have found someone who is helping with home deliveries (or who has the necessary skills and might be persuaded to help you), it is a good idea for you and your partner to meet with her or to invite her to your house for dinner. Find out who she is—what her experience is, what her attitude is, what her procedures are—and let her find out who you are. If it is a doctor who has a homebirth practice, you may have to make an appointment for an interview first. Get to know each other so you can both decide if it is appropriate for you to be working together.

Of course, your prospective birth attendant will also be getting to know you, too. And she may even decide, for whatever reason, that she doesn't want to be working with you. It can be quite discouraging, after finally locating a potential source of aid, to have her not come through or refuse you. But in fact, if a birth attendant does not want to work with you, you are better off not working with her.

The following points certainly can't all be covered in a single meeting (don't give her the third degree!), but

prior to your delivery you should know the following about your attendant.

1. *Training and Experience.*

What training has she had? How much home and hospital experience? What is her orientation toward birth? (Has she ever apprenticed with a midwife? Why does she do home deliveries?)? How many births has she attended, and at how many was she the primary attendant? There are differences between a friend with some birth experience, someone who has caught ten babies, and someone who has caught 100, 350 or 3000. Some sources say that your birth attendant should have had experience at some minimum number of births, but I feel that, rather than relying solely on numbers, you should gain a realistic appraisal of this person's level of experience (as well as an intuitive estimation of her ability to act with calm and clarity in any situation) and evaluate her skills against what you feel are the risks and what you feel you need from a birth attendant.

2. *Complications and Emergencies.*

Find out what complications and emergencies she has seen, and how they were dealt with. Find out what she can handle at home. She should be able to recognize danger signs and know what is beyond her ability. What would she do if you were bleeding and went into shock? What would she do if the baby was born white and limp and didn't start to breathe? Can she do suturing? Get a realistic idea of her areas of competency and inexperience.

3. *Medical Backup.*

If your birth attendant is an M.D. or osteopath, does he have hospital privileges? If a midwife, does she have a doctor whom she can call with questions or who will meet you at the hospital? If not, you should have your own backup (through prenatal care) and/or be familiar with the emergency room procedures of your hospital (see Emergency Backup, p. 50). Will she be able to accompany you and serve as consumer advocate at the hospital, or does she need to leave you once you are on your way to the doctor's or hospital? Does she have a pediatrician for backup (or do you)?

4. *Equipment.*

What equipment does she bring? She should have a fetoscope, bulb syringe for suctioning the baby, cord clamps or ties (or hemostats for emergencies), a disinfecting agent for scrubbing up, and sterile gloves. What does she expect you to have on hand? What emergency equipment does she bring: Oxygen? Ergotrate tablets or

methergin or pitocin to handle postpartum hemorrhage? Any other herbs or medications? Does she bring
a scale for weighing the baby? Does she have silver
nitrate or Ilotycin for the baby's eyes?

5. *Procedures.*

Does she bring an assistant? Some doctors and midwives have a very medical view of birth and bring lots
of equipment (see Seth's birth account). When does she
cut the cord? Will she let your husband assume an active role in the delivery if that's what you want? In what
capacity are you having her be present: To advise you if
anything is wrong? To actually deliver the baby? If you
want to use the LeBoyer's or other special means of welcoming your baby, does she understand and is she in
agreement? What percentage of the women she works
with tear and require stitching?

6. *Fees.*

What does her fee include? Do you think it is reason-
able? When does she want payment, and is it to be in
cash or supplies or some kind of trade? What if she
doesn't make it to the birth? What if you end up having
to go to the hospital? If the fee includes prenatal care,
delivery and six-week checkup, it should be quality prenatal care as described in Chapter Two. If she does not
provide her own prenatal care, she should be involved
with your records and lab results and should meet with
you several times prior to the birth. When does she want
to be notified and when does she come during labor?
Does she visit you in the days following the birth? How
much is she willing to invest in you and your well-
being?

7. *Communication.*

Communicate with her about who you are and what
you expect from a birth attendant. Some birth attendants are encouraged by the fact that you are taking responsibility and wouldn't agree to be there under any
other conditions; others who are used to being in charge
may want a more "professional" relationship.

   Also try to feel how open and willing she is to communicate with you, now and during labor and delivery.
How involved will she be in your labor, or will she be
primarily focusing on the birth? See how willing she is
to explain things to you, to help you see the conse-
quences of your choices, but to let you make your own
decisions. Does she teach childbirth preparation classes
or recommend someone with whom you can work?

   If she is bringing an assistant, can you get to know
her as well? It's also important that all of the people
who will be present meet with your attendant(s) and
with each other to get to know one another and so you
can discuss what is important to you. Share this book
with your attendant so she understands part of your
preparation.

8. *Attitude.*

What is her attitude toward birth? Does her attitude
mesh with yours? Is she warm, confident and caring?
Does her spiritual orientation mesh with yours? Do you
like her and feel good about her participating in your
birth?

   You won't be able to find the *ideal* birth attendant
(the one of your best imaginings). Instead you will find
real men and women who are concerned with the quality of birth and are, either tentatively or boldly, helping
with homebirths. The more you can communicate with
your attendant, the better friends you will become, and
the fewer surprises you are likely to have at the birth
itself.

IF YOU PLAN A HOSPITAL BIRTH

Since it can be difficult and costly to interview doctors,
try to find those who are the most sympathetic to true
natural childbirth by talking to childbirth educators
and La Leche League mothers. Don't feel that you have
to be content with whomever your insurance gives you.
Remember that you are hiring a doctor and have a right
to change doctors at any point during your pregnancy,
even in labor.

   When interviewing a doctor, ask questions that will
yield specific answers, like: How many of your clients
have a fetal monitor during labor? What percentage
deliver without an episiotomy?

   Once you have a doctor with whom you find you
can communicate, formulate a birth plan listing the
things that are important to you and the agreements
you have made. Detailed suggestions are included in
Pregnant Feelings.[1] In general you will probably want
to avoid unnecessary procedures such as shaving the
pubic hair and an enema, and "just in case" procedures
that can actually compromise the labor and health of a
healthy mother and baby. These would include anything that hampers your position, such as an IV drip, an
electronic fetal monitor, or stirrups. If you eat and
drink during labor, you won't need a glucose drip, and
your baby's heart tones can be monitored with a regular fetoscope. This leaves you free to walk, sit and squat,
positions that work with gravity, shorten labor and help
to open the pelvis.

   You should be aware that painkilling drugs (injections of Demerol or spinal anesthesia) are freely offered

---

[1]See Chapter Eight of *Pregnant Feelings* by Rahima Baldwin and
Terra Palmarini (Berkeley, CA: Celestial Arts, 1986).

in the hospital. Demerol makes you fuzzy and less able to cope with contractions. All drugs cross the placenta, and a normal amount of spinal anesthesia for a pregnant woman is a tremendous dose for an eight-pound infant with an immature liver to clear from its system. Your resolve to avoid drugs is best for your baby and prevents complications like fetal distress or the need for forceps, since you can't push the baby out when you're numb. After the hard work of labor, having a spinal for the exciting work of pushing means you become passive and miss all the sensations and the exhilaration of giving birth.

You can request that an episiotomy (cutting the birth canal) *not* be done. If your doctor insists, you can arm yourself with studies cited in *Episiotomy and the Second Stage of Labor* by Kitzinger and Simkin.[2] Your doctor may well not know how to do perineal support for the birth of the head without tearing, but some midwives feel it is better to tear along a place that is naturally weak than to have both a scar and the same weak place in a future birth. If you must have an episiotomy, request that it be done only after the head is well down on the perineum and stretching the skin very thin. Then most of the blood is out of the tissues and the nerve endings are deadened from the pressure of the baby's head. You can even have an episiotomy without any local anesthesia at that point, and the cut will be far smaller than the gashes made earlier in second stage.

You will also want to think about requests for the baby—such as nursing as soon as possible, no separation, newborn exam done in your presence, no supplemental bottles of sugar water, rooming in, or early dismissal. You also need to consider issues such as vitamin K and circumcision, which will be discussed later in this book.

Plan to tour the birth center or maternity ward of the hospital you will be using. The more familiar something is, the less frightening it will be. Also take care of pre-admission paper work so there will be no need for you and your partner to be separated.

If you will not be birthing with midwives, it is especially recommended that you have a labor assistant as well as your husband to be with you in the hospital. A labor assistant is a woman who is familiar with childbirth and who can support you and your husband during labor, reassuring you that everything is all right, reminding you of your resolves, and mediating between you and hospital staff should that be necessary. In the case of complications she can provide a more objective view, remind you that you can ask for a second opinion, and go a long way toward preventing unnecessary cesareans.

A child birth assistant can be a trained professional, a childbirth educator, or a knowledgeable friend. Her role can be as active or as invisible as you want it to be. You should get to know her just as you would a midwife, being clear about her views of birth and about what you want. You will want someone who will let you make your own decisions, not force her own views on you. Sometimes couples fear that another person will get in the way of their experience together, but childbirth assistants are usually very sensitive to helping strengthen the family relationship, and the presence of a woman who really knows birth can be very reassuring. It's hard for a husband who has attended six weeks of childbirth preparation classes to know if something is really all right or if you're really doing fine. And it's hard for him to provide eye contact and pressure on your sacrum for back labor at the same time! For a detailed discussion of the role and value of the labor assistant, see *Silent Knife: Cesarean Prevention and Vaginal Birth after Cesarean.*[3]

NO PRAISE AND NO BLAME

Many times throughout this book I stress the importance of parents maintaining responsibility for their own birth, and of not entering into a dependent relationship with their birth attendant, their pediatrician, or whomever. More than this, I advocate a sense of friendship, trust and unity among all the people present at a birth. If this is maintained, there will be the sense of a group of people united in a common effort, each contributing what he or she has to offer, all participating in a group process which is unique to that moment.

This shared sense of everyone doing his or her best, combined with the recognition of the uniqueness and non-repeatability of each situation, could, I am convinced, go a long way towards eliminating the aura of fear, blame and guilt which is unfortunately so prevalent in our health-care system today. It might reduce the fear of lawsuits, censure, and astronomical malpractice insurance which keeps many doctors from being involved in homebirth and leads to such a high cesarean rate in our hospitals.

Likewise, the recognition of the uniqueness of each situation should help to keep us from comparing, from saying, "If only I'd had my baby in the hospital" or "If only I'd had my baby at home." The woman who says, "I hemorrhaged after the birth in the hospital. If I'd been at home, I would have died" doesn't realize that had she been doing a homebirth, the situation would have been completely different (e.g., she wouldn't have

---

[2]Sheila Kitzinger and Penny Simkin, *Episiotomy and the Second Stage of Labor* (Seattle, WA: Pennypress, rev. 1984).

[3]See Chapter 11 of *Silent Knife* by Nancy Cohen and Lois Estner (South Hadley, MA: Bergin and Garvey, 1983).

had any drugs, her birth attendant would have been different, delivery of the placenta would have been managed differently, etc.). The same is true when some difficulty arises at home. It's impossible to say whether it or some other situation would have arisen in a hospital delivery; everything would have been different.

In making the decision to be alive and have a baby, you are admitting that there are no guarantees, either at home or in the hospital. Life is an inherently risky venture into the unknown. You can reduce risks as much as possible by being as responsible as you can. And whomever you ask to help you, whether an obstetrician, a midwife or a group of friends, you must know that all the people present are sharing and doing their best, based on their experience and their ability to be aware (and to keep each other aware), and that the "results" are dependent on something higher than ourselves, and hence go beyond praise or blame for the individuals involved.

PLANNING YOUR EMERGENCY BACKUP

Unless you can find someone who is able to give you continuity of care (prenatal, home delivery, and hospital privileges), you will also need to think about what you will do in case your delivery is among the small percentage requiring hospital care. It's important to think about these things now, so in case of an emergency you will have worked out all of the details and can quickly get the help you need.

It is helpful if your birth attendant has hospital privileges, or is a midwife with her own doctor, but you should still go through the following two pages so you will have all the information you need should your birth attendant not make it to the birth on time. Most homebirths proceed without incident, but being responsible means having considered all of the possibilities.

To help you with your emergency backup plan, fill in the following worksheet, and then fill in the numbers you will want to have posted by your telephone, and tape them to the wall *a month before your due date*.

EMERGENCY NUMBERS
TO BE POSTED BY YOUR PHONE

Name and phone numbers of birth attendants: _____

_____

_____

Name and numbers of others to be called when labor begins: _____

_____

_____

Name and number of doctor providing backup: _____

Number of emergency room of hospital: _____

   Of admissions dept.: _____

Paramedics: _____

Private ambulance service: _____

Pediatrician's name and number: _____

24-hour pharmacy: _____

EMERGENCY BACKUP WORKSHEET

FINDING A DOCTOR:

With whom have you been receiving prenatal care? _____

Will he help with the delivery? _____

Does he have hospital privileges? Where? _____

If not coming to the house, do you have a doctor who will meet you at the hospital in case of emergency? (name and phone:) _____

If you are having a midwife help you, does she have a doctor who will provide backup? _____

CHECK THE HOSPITALS IN YOUR AREA:

Which handle obstetrics? _____

Does the emergency room have an obstetrician on duty or on call? _____

Would they take you in case of an emergency? _____

(Private hospitals often do not have to take emergency cases that don't already have a private doctor there. Sometimes they can send you on to a county, or otherwise publicly funded, hospital).

Ask if there are ever maternity tours (monthly, or with Lamaze classes). The more familiar something is, the less intimidating.

Private or smaller hospitals may have the advantage of being less impersonal; a large teaching hospital might be better for an emergency cesarean or other major complication.

CHECK THE PARAMEDICS IN YOUR AREA:

Do they have training in emergency childbirth? _____

What equipment do they bring? _____

Will they take you where you want to go, or are they required to take you to the *nearest* hospital? _____

Are they contacted through the fire, police or sheriff's departments, and do these officers accompany them on a call? _____

Is there a fee? _____

CHECK THE PRIVATE AMBULANCE SERVICES:

Will they come to where you live? _____

Will they take you where you want to go, or only to the nearest hospital? _____

What is their fee? _____ Required in advance? _____

Any other requirements? _____

LINING UP A PEDIATRICIAN

Although well-baby clinics, which are either free or very low in cost, can provide most of the health care a normal child will need, there are advantages to contacting a pediatrician during your pregnancy. If you have to deliver in the hospital, you will need a pediatrician to examine the baby before checking out, and if you require a cesarean, a pediatrician will take charge of the baby at the birth. In both cases it is better to have someone you have chosen rather than a randomly selected doctor. Also, if the baby has problems, a doctor who already knows you is more likely to be willing to see and take care of the baby on short notice.

Talk to breastfeeding mothers for recommendations on good pediatricians. Some questions you should ask a prospective pediatrician include:

What is his attitude towards breastfeeding? _____

Towards supplementary bottles and introducing solid foods? _____

Towards homebirth? _____

Where does he have hospital privileges? _____

Will he come to the house after the baby is born? _____

Which hospitals in your area have neonatal intensive care units? _____

RESOURCES IN YOUR COMMUNITY

One of the best ways of preparing for your birth is by attending classes taught by an Informed Homebirth/Informed Birth and Parenting instructor if they are available in your community. You can write to the national office for the name of the instructor nearest you. If none are available, you will do better to take childbirth preparation classes from an independent instructor rather than someone who works for a doctor or the hospital. Such instructors tend to be more consumer-oriented and are free to speak for alternatives. Types of childbirth preparation are discussed in Chapter Six. You may also want to purchase the Informed Homebirth Tape Series of six cassettes that was made to accompany this book and provide further information on preparing for a home birth.

The best way to find resources is on your local level (hospitals or doctor's offices can usually give you names of childbirth educators and La Leche League leaders), but I have included the following list of national organizations which can often provide contacts in your area or can send you other useful information.

American Academy of Husband-Coached Childbirth
P.O. Box 5224
Sherman Oaks, California 91413
(Classes in the Bradley Method of childbirth preparation, teacher training, film rentals)

American College of Home Obstetrics
2821 Rose St.
Franklin Park, Illinois 60131
(Doctors in homebirth practice)

American College of Nurse-Midwives
1522 K Street, NW, Suite 1000
Washington, DC 20005

American Society for Psychoprophylaxis in Obstetrics (ASPO)
1101 Connecticut Ave., Suite 300
Washington, DC 20036
(Classes in the Lamaze Method of childbirth preparation)

Association for Childbirth at Home International (ACHI)
P.O. Box 39498
Los Angeles, CA 90039
(Homebirth classes, referrals, leder training)

Association of Labor Assistants and Childbirth   C)
Educators (ALACE), P.O. Box 382724,Cambridge,
MA 02238
(homebirth educators and labor assistants)   n)

International Cesarean Awareness Network (ICAN),
P.O. Box 276, Clark's Summit, PA 18411

Informed Homebirth/Informed Birth and Parenting
P.O. Box 3675
Ann Arbor, MI 48106
(Rahima Baldwin Dancy, President. Books, cassettes, videos, referrals and other resources. Developed the childbirth educator and birth assistant training programs now run by ALACE.)

International Childbirth Education Association (ICEA)
P.O. Box 20048
Minneapolis, MN 55420
(Prepared childbirth classes; teacher training, conferences)

La Leche League International (LLLI)
9616 Minneapolis Ave.
Franklin Park, Illinois 60131
(Monthly meetings about breastfeeding, help with difficulties)

Midwives' Alliance of North American (MANA),
P.O. Box 175
Newton, KS 67114
(Referrals, newsletter, studies, conferences)

National Association of Parents and Professionals for
    Safe Alternatives in Childbirth
    (NAPSAC)
Rt. 1, Box 646
Marble Hill, Missouri 63764
(Referrals, studies, newsletter, conferences)

Waterbirth International, P.O. Box 1400, Wilsonville, OR 97070
(Books, Videos and other resources)

OTHER GROUPS OFFERING SUPPORT, SUPPLIES, ETC.

ALACE Book Store, P.O. Box 382724, Cambridge, MA 02238
Books and videos on alternatives in birth.

Cascade Birthing Supplies Center
P.O. Box 12203
Salem, OR 97309
Full range of cord clamps, fetoscopes, other medical supplies.

Children and Hospitals
31 Wilshire Park
Needham, Massachusetts 02192
Offering information and support on the options available when babies and children need to be hospitalized. Working for change in hospitals.

Directory & Consumer Guide to Alternative Birth
Complete Mother, P.O. Box 209, Minot, ND 58702,
   Quarterly Journal Support breastfeeding and natural
mothering.

NAPSAC
Rt. 1, Box 646
Marble Hill, Missouri 63764
   Valuable national directory. Call (314) 238-2010 for
ordering information.

ICEA Book Store
Box 20048
Minneapolis, Minnesota 55420
   Write for "Bookmarks", which reviews and offers
books and other supplies for sale. They also have a cata-
logue of childbirth films available for sale or rental.

Midwifery Today
P.O. Box 2672
Eugene, OR 97402
   Outstanding quarterly magazine on birth and
midwifery.

Mothering Magazine
P.O. Box 1690
Sante Fe, New Mexico 87504
   Excellent quarterly magazine.

Birth Gazette
42, The Farm
Summertown, Tennessee 38483
   $25/year. Quarterly journal published by The Farm
to link midwives all over the world.

SUPPLIES FOR A HOMEBIRTH

WHERE TO FIND SUPPLIES

All of your supplies should be together a month in advance. Most of the items mentioned here can be found
at local drug or discount department stores. Fetoscopes
cost about $30 from medical supply stores or mail order
companies listed above.

A WORD ABOUT STERILE TECHNIQUE

Most homes are clean enough, and you are sufficiently
immune to your own germs that you don't need the ster-
ility of the hospital delivery room. Also, you aren't dealing with a succession of women delivering in your bed,
different shifts of nurses coming and going, the danger
of staph infections, and so on. *However,* it is important
that anything that goes into the mother's vagina or is involved in cutting the baby's cord be sterile (i.e., free
from any living micro-organisms) to prevent infection
in the mother or baby.

   During labor you can sterilize scissors, cord clamps
or ties by placing them in a pan of water that is already
boiling and leaving them at a boil for at least twenty
minutes. Remove with tongs and place in a casserole
with lid, and cover with alcohol. If the bulb syringe is
sealed in plastic, it is probably clean enough; otherwise
boil it for 45 minutes and let it cool, wrapping it with
gauze (do not place in alcohol).

   It is not necessary to sterilize baby clothes, but it can
be done by wrapping them in a paper bag after they
have been washed and dried. Place the bag in the oven
at 250° for one hour; put a pan of water on another
shelf to maintain moisture. Store in a plastic bag.

HOMEBIRTH SUPPLIES LIST

Sterile Pack
4x4 sterile gauze squares for perineal support.
Cord clamps: 2 plastic or metal clamps or hemostats; a
new white cotton shoe lace cut in half will do adequately.
Bulb syringe: 3-oz. ear syringe for suctioning baby.
Sharp scissors with a blunt point for cutting the cord.
Sterile disposable gloves: at least six pairs.

Clean Linen
Sheets for labor and delivery and afterwards.
Baby clothes and receiving blankets.
Towels for shower after delivery; wash cloths.
Plastic sheet (shower curtain or drop cloth) to put under
the sheets to protect mattress.
Disposable pads to put underneath mother: "Chux" by
Johnson & Johnson; or large disposable diapers.

Equipment to Borrow
Fetoscope
Blood pressure cuff and meter
Oxygen

Equipment for Labor
Betadine solution: to use on hands after scrubbing and
on mother before exams.
Rubbing alcohol.
Fleet enema to use if needed.
Unopened bottle of olive oil for perineal massage.

Tongs for sterile equipment or hot compresses.

Large bowl for placenta.

Ice bag; ice chips.

Heating pad or hot water bottle.

Soups, blender drinks, juices.

Flashlight for watching for placenta and tears.

Camera with high speed film; tape recorder if desired.

The room should be clean, with good lighting and a way to darken it if you want dim light on a bright day.

Plastic baby bath for the LeBoyer technique, if desired.

Large mirror so the mother can see.

MORE SUPPLIES FOR THE IMMEDIATE POSTPARTUM PERIOD

For the Mother
Sanitary pads and belt (hospital-size).

Thermometer.

Betadine (to mix with water and have by the toilet to pour over the genital area for tears or stitches).

DermaPlast, herbal compresses or aloe vera if you are sore from tearing/stitches.

Juices! Drink a lot after the birth and every time you nurse. Also good to have some prune juice to avoid constipation during the first few days.

Nursing bras: Not too tight, cotton lined, and able to be opened with one hand. You will definitely need to have them on hand when your milk comes in.

Pure lanolin, aloe vera or cocoa butter for sore nipples.

For the Baby
Alcohol for cord care

Baby clothes (try to get natural fibers):

3–6 undershirts, 2–4 kimonos, 4–6 nightgowns or babysuits, 2 pairs booties and 1 sweater (if winter), 4–6 receiving blankets, several newborn hats.

Cloth diapers, pins and wool soakers or rubber pants; disposable diapers (watch for diaper rash from rubber, paper or detergent)

Crib sheets; rubberized pads for changing the baby

HOSPITAL BIRTH SUPPLIES LIST

For the Mother
Nightgown or pajamas

Robe and slippers

Toothbrush and toothpaste

Shampoo, comb and brush

Underclothes and nursing bras

T-shirt or smock to wear in labor (if you wish)

Warm socks for labor

Comfort items for labor, such as massage oil, baby powder, chapstick, something for back pressure if desired, snacks that will keep, your own pillows, pictures, etc.

Camera and/or tape recorder, film, tapes, batteries

Phone numbers and coins for pay phone

Comfortable clothes if you'll be staying a few days (remember, you're not sick!), reading and writing material

Going home clothes (same size as five-months pregnant)

For the Baby
One set of baby clothes (see above)

Infant car seat

Bring a large suitcase with you, as you will take home more than you bring. The hospital will provide you with:

Ice chips, juice, soda, ice cream

Wash cloths, towels and soap

Sanitary napkins and belt

Nursing pads

Diapers and clothes for baby

Lots of free samples (make pancakes with the Similac)

PREPARATION CHECKLIST

At the beginning of your last month of pregnancy, check your preparation for the birth. The following are all things to do, but one of the most important things is your confidence, attitude and intuition about how the birth will go.

☐ Copy of prenatal records; no contra-indications to the homebirth.

☐ Know what your hematocrit is: _____

☐ Sure about where you will be living (try not to move the month before or after the birth!).

☐ Have met with your primary birth attendant several times.

☐ Decided who will be attending the birth; gotten everyone together at your house.

☐ Posted all emergency numbers by your phone.

- [ ] Assembled all supplies for the birth and immediate postpartum period.
- [ ] Your partner has read this book.
- [ ] You've both done other reading on homebirth.
- [ ] Attended homebirth classes if available (or used the tapes).
- [ ] Feel confident about being able to breathe, relax and deliver the baby (attended classes and/or practiced together as a couple).
- [ ] Attended La Leche League meetings or have books on hand to answer questions during the first week of breastfeeding.

- [ ] Listened to your baby's heart tones (they are _____/minute).
- [ ] Know the route to the hospital (have a map marked if necessary).
- [ ] Know where the emergency entrance is.
- [ ] Have both practiced CPR on a doll (See Ch. 8; if possible, take a course in CPR from your local Red Cross).
- [ ] You both know how to do bi-manual pressure on the uterus for hemorrhage (See Ch. 8).

THE BIRTHS OF CHISPA *(Spark)* AND MARIPOSA *(Butterfly)*

Margaret and Jenny Fiedler

Margaret writes:

Birth is creation itself. It is also a metaphor for creation: to know that I am only the channel through which a new being passes from one state to another is, simultaneously, to know that without the channel there is no passage. I am, as a mother, at the same time totally dispensable (life does not come *from* me, but *through* me) and totally indispensable.

When a group of us, eleven Mexicans and Americans living together in Cuernavaca, Mexico, in 1973, decided to study midwifery, it was not because we wanted to become midwives nor was it even because two of the group (who happened to be the two youngest of my six children) were pregnant. We were looking for a new way of living, of being, which would not turn love into hate. We decided to study (and be) the birthing process as a model for a whole new way of learning, of loving, of getting to know ourselves. At the time, however, we had very little idea of either the power or the inevitability of what we were doing.

In fact, our first idea was that all we had to do was to decondition ourselves. (I am using the words as we used them then.) Our intention was to support one another and to retain our own power, rather than giving it over to credentialized "authorities." Regarding the births, we saw that having the daring and strength to trust ourselves rather than turning to an expert was the manifestation of an inner change in consciousness for us all. At that point we thought we could just act naturally—just have a baby.

What we discovered, however, is that there is nothing simple or unconscious about acting "natural-ly." All wisdom, it turns out, is conscious wisdom. The romantic notion that (so-called) primitive women just squat in the fields and have their babies, sling them on their backs and go back to work, is just that: a romantic notion. The truth is that birth, like all aspects of life, including death, is always our own creation; every culture has its gospel, its Way. Truth is One, but there are ten thousand ways of knowing the One. It is only my ignorance of someone else's understanding that allows me to assume they do something "by accident" or by "good luck" or "simply."

How does this apply to what happened to us then, and to what is happening at so many births today? Having taken responsibility for ourselves, we found that acting naturally doesn't "come naturally." So we decided that we must each become an expert, learn everything about births. Then it came to us that to do this would be to fall off the tightrope on the other side. I see this happening in the homebirth movement today. It is becoming over-medicalized (if the heartbeat is such and such, get thee to a hospital, instead of listening to the vibrations). It is becoming defensive ("We're just as sterilized in our humble trailer as you are in your sterile hospital"). It is becoming judgmental ("She's a good midwife because she has attended a certain number of births").

We came to realize that birth is an integral part of the continuum of life, not a series of separate emergencies. There is a saying in the East, "Trust in God, but tether your camel." Don't worry about what you will tether your camel with—anything that comes to hand, anything that comes to mind, anything that comes to consciousness. If you are thinking in terms of progress, of getting a better rope, of learning a better way to tether your camel, you have lost your trust in God.

Creation, birth does not wait. How silly to say, "Wait! Stop, until I have learned to do it better." Either I am prepared, right here and now, to do the best I can, or I am not alive at all, am not creating or created, am letting someone else do it, letting someone else be instead of *my* being.

All of this, and lots more, is what we explored in the group that we sometimes called "The Birthday Party." In some ways it could be seen as the survival groping of an endangered species.

Jenny writes:

Memo, my sister, went into labor first. I was nervous, but she was incredibly calm. The whole group breathed together with each contraction. None of us had been at a homebirth before, much less done one. In trying to check dilation, we didn't really know what to feel for, so we drew pictures for each other and talked about how the cervix felt.

After thirty hours of heavy labor, Memo still wasn't fully dilated. She was still completely relaxed and in control when Margarita began to suspect that the baby was breech and we decided to go to someone with more experience.

We went driving around Cuernavaca. One midwife checked Memo and said the baby *was* breech, but she didn't want to do the delivery. Memo was still breathing through contractions and was relaxed and happy. Finally we found a doctor who told us he would deliver the baby in the hospital, by cesarean if necessary, and with none of us present. Yikes!

Memo rode with him in his car from his office to the hospital. The rest of us followed. By the time we got to the hospital Memo had radicalized him—she was so calm and wonderful. He didn't do a cesarean, but reached in with his hands, using no drugs, and delivered Chispa breech. He was a perfect, cute little boy—thank God! Memo and Bob and Chispa rested in the hospital for a few hours and came home that evening, March 25, 1974, after a 34-hour labor.

Somehow I had gotten it in my head that since we'd been pregnant together, we would have the babies together. So the next three weeks before I went into labor seemed so long!

To discuss Posy's birth, I'd like to include what I wrote then, in April 1974.

"Mariposa—my sweet Butterfly—you came flying out of me Thursday afternoon, still wrapped in your white cocoon (the creamy vernix). Tears start to flow out of me as I think about it—I'm still so full of you.

"When I woke up Thursday, I couldn't believe the water that came out of me was your beginnings. So anxious for you to come, so eager not to make you feel hur-

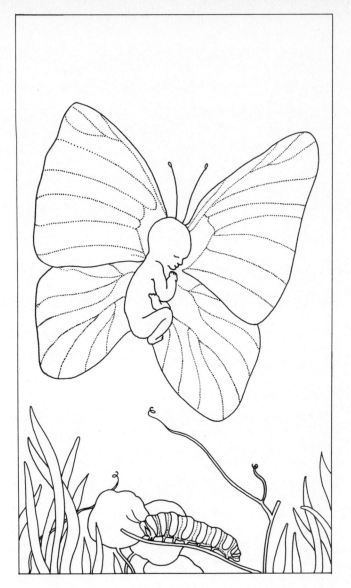

FIGURE 4-1.

ried. But it was you, and contractions started. I could see my stomach dance with your eagerness to get out. I went to my bed, with all the family surrounding me except Sergio, who was still at work. The minute the contractions started, I was totally at peace. You were sending me messages that everything was fine. All my worries or fears were gone, and I was totally relaxed into our job of getting you out.

"Everybody was so with me, each knowing his or her job, finding it and doing it. Sergio came at noon, and you were only three hours from coming. When you started, you were in a hurry to do it!

"I felt Sergio's hand on my wrist, pouring all his love and strength into me. Everyone was scurrying to find warm socks for me, taking pictures, boiling water; I was floating and breathing and breathing, with everyone stopping everything to breathe with me.

"Then it was time to push—a confusing moment—and then it was together. You came so fast that with each push everyone could see more of your head. I saw it with a mirror, and I couldn't believe you would be in the world in a few minutes. I was shaking with the effort of working you out.

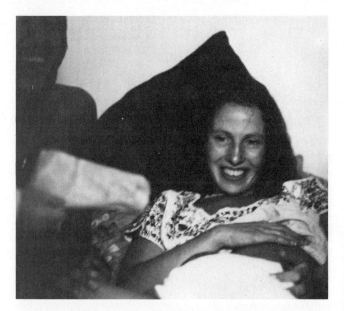

FIGURE 4-2. *Relaxing in labor, surrounded by friends.*

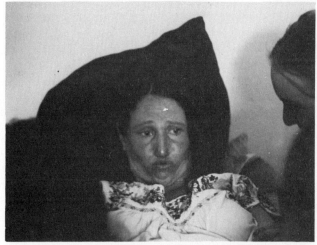

FIGURE 4-4. *"What is pushing, anyway?"*

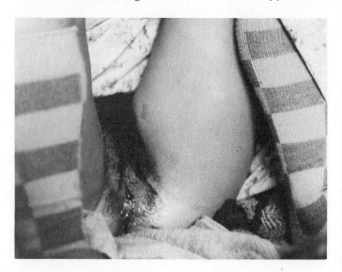

FIGURE 4-3. *Bloody show of active labor. Warm socks help the chills!*

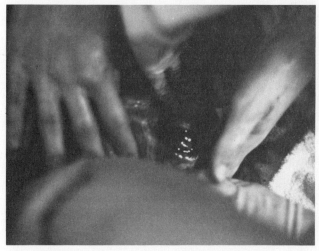

FIGURE 4-5. *Posy's head beginning to show.*

"My first transition contraction was amazing. Patty was sitting between my legs . . . Bob and Margarita holding my feet . . . Memo and Sergio my wrists . . . they were all part of me. Without all my parts I couldn't have done it . . . Billy's pictures . . . Debby's loving tears . . . Barbara's presents . . . Paul's touch . . . Tal's wide eyes . . . Lisa's flower . . . Janet's confused fear, love, pain and sharing . . . and even Arnie's ice cream. I felt stoned. Everyone had halos around them.

"It was so hard to know what to do. Push? Wait? What is pushing, anyway? Memo was tuned in so completely, breathing and talking, giving me instructions. *I* was so much the job of getting you out, that nothing else existed. It felt like Memo's voice was coming from inside me. With each contraction I would look into everyone's eyes, everyone so with me and yet so much themselves.

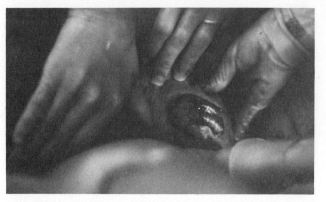

FIGURE 4-6. *Support and massage as the head stretches the perineum.*

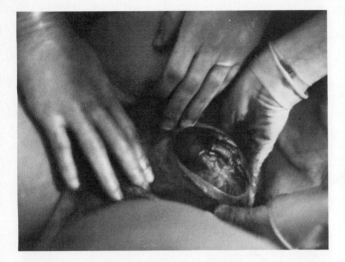

FIGURE 4-7. *The head crowns . . .*

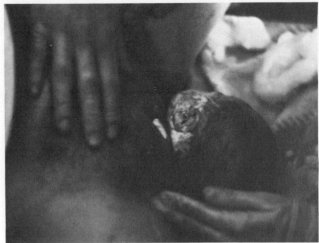

FIGURE 4-9. *The head turns toward the side.*

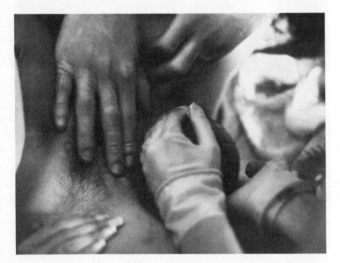

FIGURE 4-8. *. . .and is born!*

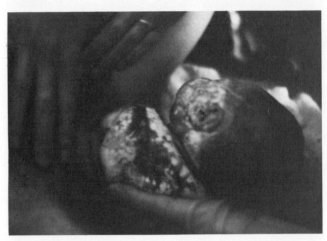

FIGURE 4-10. *The shoulders and the rest of the baby follow quickly!*

"All of a sudden your head crowned, and Patty started shaking, realizing she was where you were coming out. Bob helped her stretch the perineum so it wouldn't rip. Your head was out!

"One minute later you came flooding, flowing, gushing out, all covered in your white cocoon, into Patty's arms: your tongue out, one eye open, breathing. Shining eyes all around—tears and smiles. There you were in the world, my Butterfly, my Mariposa.

"I tied your cord, still shaking. Margarita cut it. Patty sucked the mucus from your mouth. Sergio, Bob and Raoul buried the placenta.

"My beautiful friend—none of us could believe how big you were—bigger than Chispa who was almost a month old. We all thank you for sharing your birth with us. None of us could have done it alone!"

CHAPTER FIVE

Normal Labor and Delivery at Home

Preparing yourself to give birth involves understanding the process of labor and delivery so you know what is happening with your body, can trust your body's ability to give birth, and can correctly interpret the signals it is sending you. Fear of the unknown can cause tension, which results in discomfort and pain. In order to break that cycle, we'll explore the physiological aspects of normal labor and delivery in this chapter. In the following two chapters we'll discuss how it *feels*, and what you and your partner can do to be more comfortable and to open completely to this most exciting and rewarding of life's experiences.

WAYS IN WHICH LABOR CAN BEGIN

MUCOUS PLUG

You may discover the slightly pink, egg-white-like, mucousy substance which has kept the uterus sealed. It is often noticed when going to the toilet. It is sometimes called the *bloody show*, but shouldn't be confused with the bloody show that occurs during active labor. It is a sign that everything is getting ripe, and you will often be in labor within twenty-four hours.

BREAKING OF THE WATERS

You may miss the mucous plug and find that there is "water" (actually amniotic fluid) coming from the vagina, either by drops or in a great gush. This is a sign that the membranes have ruptured, and you should be in active labor within twenty-four hours, since once the membranes have ruptured you and the baby are open to infection. Notify your birth attendant if the waters break. Take showers only, and don't put anything in the vagina. Labor begins this way in only about ten percent of births; usually the waters don't break until around transition or second stage, when they are often accompanied by stronger, more frequent contractions.

CONTRACTIONS

This is the most common way for labor to begin, with contractions that become stronger and closer together as time goes on. If they go away after a while, or if lying down or walking around or taking a shower makes them stop, it has just been a warm-up session—a good chance to practice breathing and relaxation. In true labor the contractions will increase in intensity and the period of rest between them will decrease as labor progresses.

LABOR CONTRACTIONS

Contractions are a shortening of the muscles of the uterus which gradually cause the cervix, or muscular neck of the uterus, to become thin and to open so the baby can pass into the birth canal. The contractions push the baby down the birth canal and cause it to be born.

STAGES OF LABOR AND DELIVERY

FIRST STAGE: LABOR

Early labor (latent phase): Effacement (thinning) of the cervix. Dilation of the cervix (opening from 0 to 2½ cm). This stage can be quite long.

Active labor: Dilation from 2½ to 10 cm. Contractions become stronger and closer together. You dilate much faster.

Transition (A part of active labor.): Final dilation of the cervix (to 10 cm). It is the transition between labor and second stage. See the text for further signs of transition.

SECOND STAGE: DESCENT AND BIRTH

The baby passes through the fully-dilated cervix and down the birth canal (vagina). The mother is able to push with contractions. The head appears at the vaginal opening, crowns, and is born.

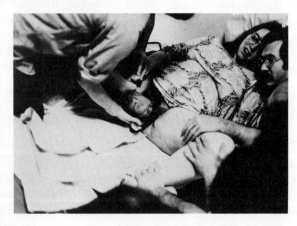

FIGURE 5-1.

THIRD STAGE: PLACENTA, OR AFTERBIRTH

The placenta (or afterbirth) comes out with the next few contractions after the birth (usually within 20 minutes). The uterus continues to contract to prevent hemorrhage. It should be massaged every 15 minutes for the first hour after the placenta is out, being felt as a hard, grapefruit sized mass below the belly button.

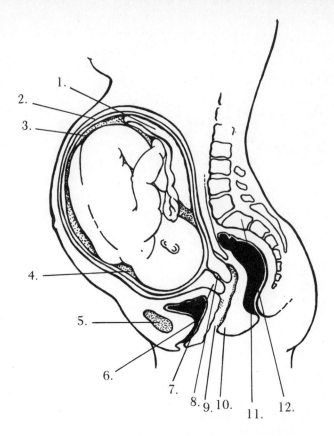

12. Spinal column.	
11. Rectum.	
10. Perineum.	
9. Vagina or birth canal.	
8. Mucous plug.	
7. Cervix.	
6. Bladder.	
5. Pubic bone.	
4. Amniotic fluid.	
3. Amniotic sac or bag of waters.	
2. Uterus.	
1. Placenta and cord.	

FIGURE 5-2. *Basic anatomy—check your knowledge by filling in the blanks.*

A contraction starts gradually, increases in intensity and gradually diminishes, forming a wave pattern. In between contractions your uterus is at rest. Contractions are often felt in the lower belly, in the back or in the thighs (in active labor your belly will feel hard to the touch during a contraction). The sensation is hard to describe to someone who has never been in labor. It is important to think of the contractions as *sensation*, rather than *pain*, which is an interpretive judgement we place on sensation. On The Farm in Tennessee, they call contractions *rushes*, which may give you a better idea of the nature of the energy involved and how to handle it.

Your uterus contracts throughout pregnancy, and you may be aware of the so-called "Braxton-Hicks contractions" during your last month or so of pregnancy. They can give you an opportunity to practice your

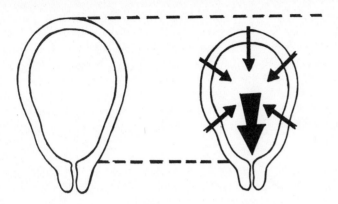

FIGURE 5-3 *Resting and contracting uterus.*

breathing and relaxation, but the contractions of labor feel quite different.

Labor may start with the mucous plug coming out or the waters breaking, but most often it starts with contractions that are fairly far apart and fairly mild. However, labor may begin with strong contractions every five minutes, especially if the waters have broken. Every labor is different, and there is no way to predict in advance how yours will be.

Labor means work, but a fifteen-hour labor doesn't mean that you're working that entire time. Like the waves of the ocean or the cycle of our breaths, labor involves contraction and release. So there is time to relax between contractions, and although the contractions do become stronger, there is usually adequate time for your body and mind to adapt to the increasing intensity.

It isn't necessary to time contractions continually, but you'll want to time them every so often to know if they are becoming more regular, and so that you can report to your birth attendant. Time contractions from the beginning of one contraction to the beginning of the next. Thus, five-minute contractions means about one minute of contraction, followed by four minutes of rest.

FIRST STAGE: LABOR

EARLY LABOR (LATENT PHASE)

Early labor is the longest phase, from the time you start feeling contractions until 2-3 centimeters dilation. You needn't think of yourself as being "in labor" all this time. In fact, the best way of dealing with early labor is to act as if it weren't happening until it demands your attention. If it is daytime, walk around, sit up and continue light activity. Being vertical increases the effectiveness of contractions. If it is night, *go back to sleep!* I know it's exciting, but don't let it turn into a slumber party and remember that you and your coach will need that extra energy at the end, especially if you have a long labor. Sleep through the first few hours; it really

can be done, and I guarantee you won't sleep through the birth!

If you get an adrenaline rush in early labor, calm down, do complete body relaxation and assess what is actually happening with your body and your contractions once you are relaxed. Everyone probably has the secret hope and fear that they will have a really short labor, but if your belly isn't rising up hard to the touch with contractions about three minutes apart, you aren't having a precipitous delivery, so continue light activity or go back to sleep. Sharing energy with your partner, hugging and kissing, is also highly recommended for early labor. The same energy that put the baby in will help to get him out, and it will put you and your partner in closer touch with each other and with the labor.

The job of early labor is the effacement and beginning dilation of the cervix. The cervix is the muscular neck of the uterus which holds the baby up and keeps everything sealed inside.

Effacement is the thinning out or taking up of the cervix through contractions. It is like putting on a turtleneck shirt: as you pull in a rhythmic fashion, simulating contractions, the neck of the shirt, which is sticking up above your head, gradually disappears as it gets pulled into the rest of the shirt.

Dilation is the opening of the cervix from 0 to 10 cm. Contractions continue to pull up the fibers of the cervix, opening it further as labor progresses.

MIDDLE OR ACTIVE LABOR

Once your cervix has opened to about 2½ cm, your dilation will proceed more rapidly from there to 4 cm (this is an accelerating phase in which the contractions and their rate of dilation are beginning to speed up). Dilation then proceeds even more rapidly from 4 cm to nearly full dilation (See Figure 5-7 on p. 64).

In order to accomplish this accelerating dilation, contractions become increasingly stronger and closer together. The period of rest between them decreases to about five minutes, then down to three minutes. Your belly will feel hard to the touch now during contractions, which will probably be about a minute long.

You'll find you are needing to concentrate more during contractions in active labor, and that you're less talkative and outgoing. Hugging and kissing with your partner can help your labor advance; stimulation of the breasts releases oxytocin, which causes the uterus to contract (nursing mothers have long known this fact, but Stephen Gaskin was the first person I know of to apply this principle to labor).

Sitting up and walking around, if you aren't too tired, can also help your labor. Relaxing in a tub of hot water can feel good now, or you may enjoy lying back, supported by lots of pillows.

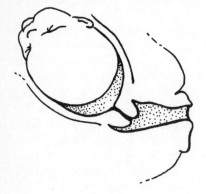
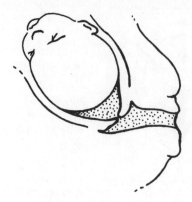
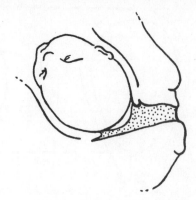

a. *As labor begins.*   b. *Effacement (cervix thinned).*   c. *Effacement with dilation.*

FIGURE 5-4. *a, b, & c*

You may get a bloody show during active labor, which is bloodier than the pinkish mucus you may have noticed before labor began. It's like menstrual bleeding, and is a good sign that labor is progressing; it is no cause for alarm. The only bleeding that is uncommon and dangerous is a bright red, stream of fresh blood coming out of the vagina. The waters may break at this time, perhaps with just a trickle from the forewaters that are in front of the baby's head, or perhaps with a gush of water with each contraction. There are one to two quarts of amniotic fluid, which all comes out sooner or later, so be prepared with a rubber sheet and disposable pads under you.

When the waters break, they should be clear and not green, brown or foul smelling; the baby's heartbeat should be monitored when the waters break to make sure the cord hasn't come down and gotten pinched. The baby's heart tones should be clear and not racing (above 170) or slow (around 100 beats per minute). The heartbeat normally slows down during a contraction, but it should quickly come back up within about five seconds after the contraction is finished and stay in the normal range between contractions. It should be listened to and written down every half hour during active labor. All equipment should be sterilized and made ready during this stage.

Early labor: contractions are perhaps a half minute long, with 5 to 30 minutes in between.

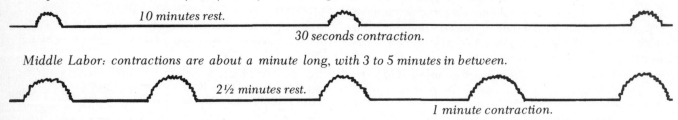

10 minutes rest.

30 seconds contraction.

Middle Labor: contractions are about a minute long, with 3 to 5 minutes in between.

2½ minutes rest.

1 minute contraction.

Transition: contractions are a minute to a minute and a half in length, with perhaps a minute in between. They are very strong, perhaps with 2 or 3 peaks, and a beginning urge to push. Transition can be rough, and require direct coaching, but it is the shortest phase and means that you'll soon be able to push.

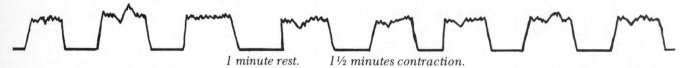

1 minute rest.   1½ minutes contraction.

Expulsion: contractions are again about a minute long, with 2-3 minutes rest in between, and you are able to push the baby out with each contraction.

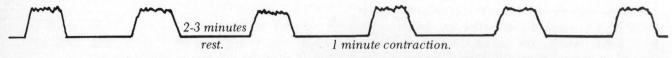

2-3 minutes rest.

1 minute contraction.

FIGURE 5-5. *As labor progresses, contractions become stronger and closer together.*

TRANSITION

Transition is the final opening of the cervix to 10 cm. In our analogy of putting on a turtleneck shirt, it is the point of maximum stretch, the time of maximum tension before the shirt slides over your head.

This final stretching of the cervix before the baby's head slips through and begins to move down the vagina (birth canal) is accompanied by contractions that are very intense and close together (perhaps a minute and a half in length, sometimes with only a minute's rest in between). They often start out strong rather than building gradually and may have two or three peaks (Figure 5-5).

You may start to feel the urge to push as the baby presses against your lower bowel, but it's important to keep breathing and not to push now. You may also experience trembling, hot and cold flashes, nausea and vomiting, or emotionality.

Transition is the most intense part of labor, but it is also the shortest. You may start getting some of the signs of transition around 7- or 8-cms dilation; but, if it is your first baby, you may still have some time to go. I call this "approaching transition." Mistakenly thinking "We only have a half hour to go" when these preliminary signs of transition arise can cause disappointment and concern, especially for first-time mothers, and even more so if your birth attendant is a bit optimistic in checking dilation.

The designation of transition according to centimeters of dilation is very imprecise and misleading, in my opinion. You would do better to neither watch for it (you may never experience the signs of it) nor be surprised by it (you may be at only 6 cm and suddenly go to full dilation in twenty minutes or less). We can say that for most women, transition is when contractions are nearly back to back, and you can't do anything but surrender to the force that is driving through your body and birthing your baby. This most intense part of labor is the shortest part, usually lasting only 30 to 45 minutes for a first baby, and perhaps 15 or 20 minutes for subsequent births, although a two-hour transition in a first-time mother is not a cause for alarm.

Direct coaching can help you most during this period, and giving out energy to your partner can also help you stay on top of contractions. You know that you will soon be into second stage and that your baby will soon be born.

If the waters haven't broken already, they will probably break in transition. The baby's heartbeat should be monitored every fifteen minutes, and it is vital to have an empty bladder in transition. You will probably feel more discomfort in your lower back as the baby's head descends lower in your pelvis. It's important not to push until dilation is complete (Figure 5-6) and the pushing urge is irresistible. For further information on handling transition, see Chapter 7.

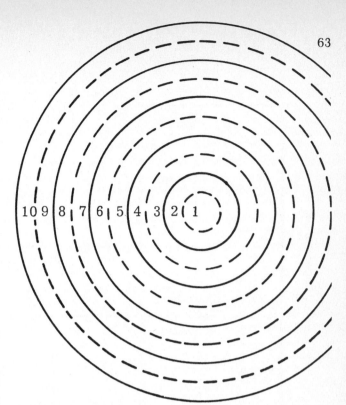

Early Labor: about 0-3 cm.   *Full dilation is usually 10*
Middle Labor: 3-7 cm.   *cm (or "five fingers"); one*
Transition: 7-10 cm.   *finger equals 2 cm.*

FIGURE 5-6. *Dilation of the cervix from 1 to 10 centimeters.*

HOW LONG DOES LABOR LAST?

Labor lasts until the baby is born. Each labor is unique—there's no way of predicting in advance. The important thing is to be in the present moment, to experience either the contraction or the rest period, and not to worry about how fast things are progressing or how long it has been. Checking dilation by having your birth attendant feel the cervix vaginally can help to mark how your labor is going, but probably the greatest single source of discouragement or of unnecessary trips to the hospital during homebirths is diagnosing the labor as being farther along than it really is and then wondering, "Where's the baby?"

If you understand certain things about the progression labor follows, it may help you to understand what is happening with your body.

The chart of Figure 5-7 was developed by physicians through averaging many women's labors. Yours may be very different without anything being wrong. Deviations from Friedman's curve are not pathological if the baby's heart tones remain good. Labor does not always progress in a smooth curve! Often there are plateaus of little progress in dilation when the baby may be turning or contractions may be less strong. But if we don't fall into the trap of expecting to conform to the average, we can notice some interesting things about the pattern of labor: that the last half of dilation is accomplished in about one-third the time. This means that even if it

Full dilation.

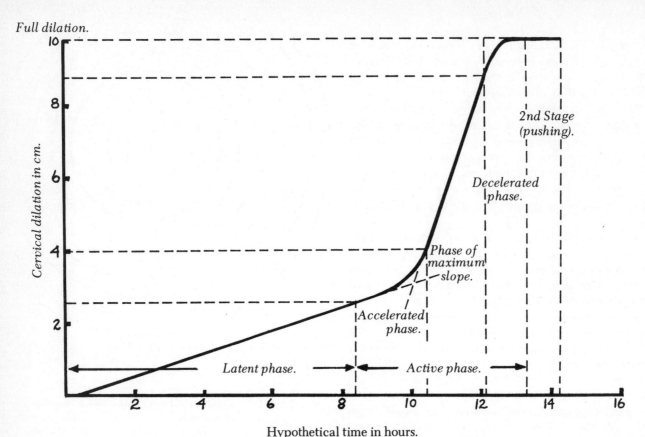

Hypothetical time in hours.
FIGURE 5-7. *As labor progresses, dilation accelerates*.*

takes you a long time to get to 2 or even 4 cms, things should move along much more rapidly after that. Don't get discouraged!

Second babies usually take less time than first babies because your body has been stretched once before. With a second or subsequent baby, the entire active phase may be only a couple of hours long; once 6-cm dilation is reached, complete dilation may follow very quickly. However, don't become discouraged if your second baby takes longer than the first; it might be in a more posterior position and have to rotate, for example.

Note also that there is a normal slowing down of progress which may occur just before dilation is complete (especially with first babies). There may be strong transition contractions without much progress if, for example, the cervix still has an anterior lip; or there may be a brief slacking off of contractions right around full dilation or just before second stage. All these are normal.

Factors that can affect how long your labor takes include individual differences, the number of previous births, your position during labor, the baby's position, the size of the baby, and psychological factors. The important thing is that progress is steady and the baby and

---

*Based on research of Emanual A. Friedman: "Use of Labor Pattern as a Management Guide," Hosp. Top., 46 (No. 8); 58, 1968.

mother are both doing well. If you are having questions about a prolonged labor (e.g., if the first stage has gone beyond 24 hours or the second stage beyond two hours), refer to the section on prolonged labor in Chapter 8.

SECOND STAGE: DELIVERY OF THE BABY

WHEN TO PUSH

Once the cervix is fully dilated, contractions will begin to push the baby down the birth canal. If you are getting a pushing urge from pressure against the rectum before you are fully dilated, it is important not to push until your cervix is completely open and the pushing urge is irresistible. Pushing too early can result in a swollen cervix, lack of progress and pain. The way to avoid pushing is to breathe through contractions: as long as you're breathing, you're not pushing.

If your birth attendant says you are fully dilated but you aren't feeling the urge to push, just keep breathing with contractions. Studies discussed in the next chapter show that you need only push when there is an irresistible urge. If your attendant is somewhat insistent, try squatting for a few contractions to see if that brings the baby down and causes a pushing urge.

Don't resist what your body is doing; don't resist the pushing *sensation* if it is there. But as long as you can breathe with contractions and the pushing urge, there is no need to add extra pushing effort to what your uterus is doing. When the contraction holds your breath involuntarily, then add pushing technique to it. Your baby can be born without a great athletic effort on your part unless something besides the vertex is presenting, or for some other reason there is lack of progress; then you may need to push vigorously, or to squat when pushing. If it hurts to push, something may be wrong: undilated cervix, malpresentation, etc. See the next chapter for a complete discussion of pushing.

DESCENT OF THE HEAD

The baby's heartbeat should be monitored every ten minutes during second stage and descent of the head noted from time to time. Descent is really a question of how far up the birth canal you have to go before encountering the baby's skull; it is measured according to the relation of the head to the ischial spines of your pelvis (when they are even, it's called 0 station; +4 or +5 is birth, Figure 5-8). The head will come down and appear at the opening during contractions, then slip back. This is the normal descent unless you are squatting: two steps down and one step back. A full bladder can impede descent and damage the bladder, so remember to urinate before second stage.

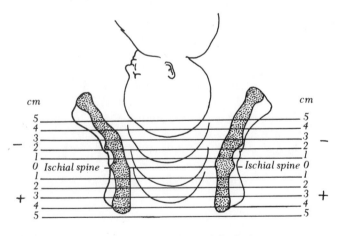

FIGURE 5-8. *Descent of the baby.*

PREVENTING TEARS

Whether or not you tear when the head comes out depends on a number of factors:

1. The condition of your tissues (good nutrition, including extra vitamins C and E, and pelvic floor exercises will help).

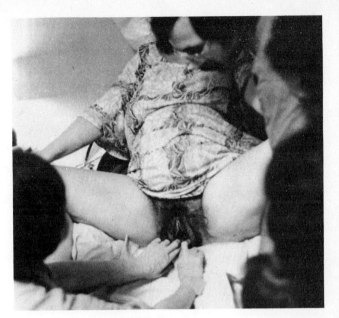

FIGURE 5-9. *Stretching the perineum with olive oil.*

2. Your position during late second stage (lying back if you've been squatting or letting the legs flop apart, rather than imitating the stirrups position, aid in the relaxation of the pelvic floor).

3. How well you are able to stop pushing when the head crowns.

4. The size and presentation of your baby.

5. The extent to which your birth attendants are able to help you with a gentle delivery of the head.

There are several things that your birth attendants can do to help you deliver without tearing. One is to apply hot compresses to your lower belly, vulva and perineum during the early part of second stage to keep the tissues supple and aid relaxation. Then once the head starts to be visible at the vaginal opening, your attendant or husband should begin to massage the perineum (the area between the vagina and anus) in between contractions. You can also massage this area yourself, both during pregnancy and during labor.

The purpose of perineal massage and support is to prevent tearing by:

1. Helping the pelvic floor muscles to relax and stretch.

2. Keeping good circulation in the perineum so it doesn't become shiny, brittle and likely to tear.

3. Supporting the perineum as the head crowns so the head doesn't come out too quickly and tear the tissues.

To massage the perineum, use pure vegetable oil (olive, avocado or almond are all good) and rub the vulva and perineal area in between contractions with small circular motions. Two fingers of each gloved hand can be inserted into the vagina, helping the muscles to relax and stretch by pressing in a downward and outward direction, enlarging the opening (Figure 5-

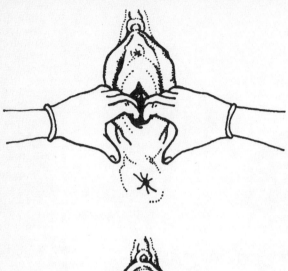

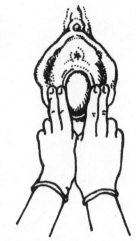

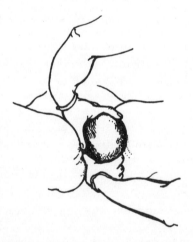

FIGURE 5-10. *(a) Stretching the vaginal opening, (b) rubbing downward, and (c) supporting the perineum.*

10a). Rubbing in a downward motion can help bring blood to the area and keep everything elastic (Figure 5-10b).

Finally, as the baby's head crowns, perineal support can be offered by means of counter pressure on the perineum. Don't push on the baby's head—gentle pressure on the mother's tissues is all that is required (Figure 5-10c). This helps the head to stay flexed and to be born without tearing the tissues.

CROWNING AND BIRTH OF THE HEAD

The head is said to be crowning when the largest diameter stretches the vaginal opening and the head doesn't slip back between contractions. It is the point of maximum tension on the perineum, and you may feel a sensation of stretching or burning, but it only lasts for a few minutes and then your baby's head slips out.

It is important when you see or feel the head crowning (or when your husband or attendant advises you) that you stop pushing so the head will not be expelled too rapidly. Light, rapid, relaxed breaths assure that only your uterus is doing the work. Perineal support should be maintained for the birth of the head.

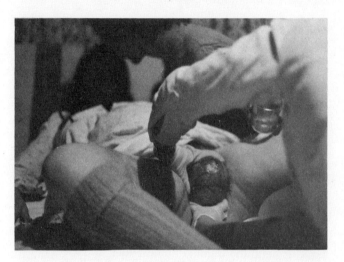

FIGURE 5-11. *A nine-pound baby born without tearing.*

When the head comes out it might be bluish in color, and is almost always face down (facing the mother's backbone). If the baby is born face up or if there is staining of the amniotic fluid, the baby should be suctioned as soon as the head is out. Otherwise it's possible to wait until the baby is out to see if he is mucousy or having trouble breathing before suctioning. Press the air out of the syringe before inserting it in the baby's mouth; release the pressure and mucus will be sucked into the syringe. Remove the syringe and squeeze/shake out the mucus. Press again, and insert into the baby's nose and suction there.

CHECKING FOR THE CORD

Once the head is out, your attendant will check for the cord around the neck (which happens in about one-third of all births). Check all the way around the neck and shoulders. Usually there is no problem if it is loose and pulsating. Most often it can be pulled up and looped over the baby's head or over the shoulders as the body is born.

It is very rare to have to cut the cord at this point.

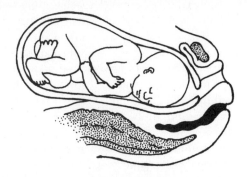

A. *Early Labor: 2 cm dilation; 80 percent effaced.*

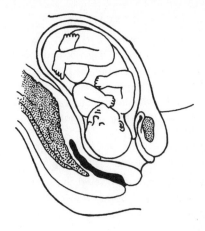

B. *Transition: 8 cm dilated; the mother should be at about a 45-degree angle; the hardest part of labor, but the shortest.*

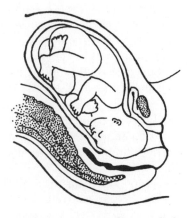

C. *Descent: Dilation is complete and the baby's head passes through the cervix and down the birth canal; the waters have usually broken; the head turns face down.*

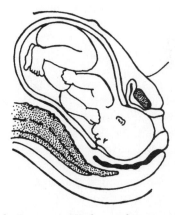

D. *Continued Descent: With each contraction, the baby's head travels further down the birth canal; the rectum becomes very compressed, causing strong pushing urges.*

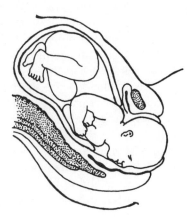

E. *Crowning: As the head crowns at the opening, the mother should stop pushing to prevent tearing of the perineum, which stretches over the baby's face as it "sweeps the perineum."*

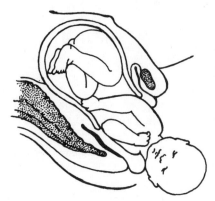

F. *Restitution: The head turns back toward the side and then the shoulders are born one at a time and the body slides out.*

FIGURE 5-12. *Labor and delivery.*

The only reason would be if the cord was around the neck twice and couldn't be unwound, or if a short cord was preventing the baby's birth or pulling on the placenta, or if the cord was so tightly around the neck that the baby was becoming congested and distressed (turning dark blue and purple, or white and limp). In these cases it should be clamped or tied in two places immediately and then cut. The baby would then need to be delivered through the mother's immediate pushing efforts, even between contractions and resuscitated if necessary (see Chapter 8). If the cord is tightly over a shoulder and being compressed, have the mother push even without a contraction and loop it over the shoulder as the body emerges to prevent strain on the placenta or umbilicus.

DELIVERY OF THE SHOULDERS

When the head comes out it is almost always face down. It need only be supported and it will turn by itself, usually toward the mother's right leg as the shoulders rotate internally in preparation for coming out. It is always amazing to have the baby half in and half out of you, and the two or three minutes between the birth of the head and the next contraction can seem like an eternity. With the next contraction, the shoulders should be born, usually (but not always) the top one first. No one should pull on the baby's head. Perineal support should be maintained to assure that the shoulders come one at a time and don't tear the perineum. If the shoulders don't come within two contractions, you should get up into a squat or on hands and knees (see Chapter 8).

Once the shoulders are out, the rest of the baby slips out, and your baby is born! Someone should record the time of birth, which is when the entire body emerges.

FOCUS ON THE BABY

BREATHING

The logical place to put the normal newborn is on the mother's belly where she can see and feel it, and where it has skin contact and the reassurance of being lovingly supported after just having been released from a tight place into the vastness of space. If it isn't warm in your room, put a warmed receiving blanket over baby and mother. Newborns don't have well-developed body temperature regulating systems and need to be kept warm.

If the baby is especially mucousy or is having trouble starting to breathe, he should be suctioned using a bulb syringe.

Babies start to breathe once their chests are free to expand (a few even take a first breath when only the head is out). The difference in temperature between even a warm room and 98.6°F is quite a drop—somewhat like jumping into a cold swimming pool—and the baby inhales just as you would. If your baby has not been drugged through maternal anesthesia and does not come out white and limp, he will start to breathe. Unless we have cleared our own birth trauma (and most of us were born under anesthesia), we tend to relive our own oxygen deprivation and have to remind ourselves to relax and breathe. If we don't we can end up with less oxygen than the baby, who still has the placental circulation to help with the transition.

If your baby comes out and has good muscle tone (arms and legs flexed or moving) and responds to touch (e.g., grimaces when suctioned), he requires only attentiveness—he will start to breathe on his own. He may start with a cry, a gasp, or just quiet gurgling noises. Allow him to find his own rhythm. If the baby is white and limp or starts to breathe and stops again, you will need to do cardiopulmonary resuscitation (see Chapter 8).

Your baby will be bluish in color until he takes the first breath; then you can see the pinkness spread from the chest area to the extremities. The head will also be molded from the birth process, but it will start to go back into shape within a few hours. For more information on the newborn, see Chapter 10.

THE APGAR SCORE

Dr. Virginia Apgar developed a series of things to look for in the newborn which were good indicators of how it was doing and whether or not it was likely to need special attention for later problems. The scoring is done, in the chart on the following page, at one minute and again at five minutes after birth:

A score of 8–10 is excellent, 4–7 is guarded, and 0–3 is critical. The score at five minutes is more significant, a low score then indicating a baby in serious condition.

The important thing is to *look at the baby*. It's not necessary to whip out your stethoscope at one minute, but really pay attention to the baby's breathing, skin color and muscle tone, its ability to respond and make the transition to an entirely different mode of existence.

CUTTING THE CORD

Once the cord has stopped pulsating (about 5 or 10 minutes), you can clamp or tie it about two inches from the baby's navel and again at three inches, then cut between the two ties. (The cord is tied in two places in case there are undiagnosed twins.)

SIGN	0	1	2	1 min. Score	5 min. Score
Heart rate	Absent	Slow (below 100)	Over 100		
Respiratory effort	Absent	Slow irregular	Good strong		
Muscle tone	Limp	Some flexion of extremities	Active motion		
Reflex irritability (response to bulb syringe or to lips being touched)	No response	Grimace	Cough or sneeze or strong grimace		
Color	Blue, Pale	Body pink, extremities blue	Completely pink		

It is important that the cord clamps or ties and your scissors be sterilized, because the cord is one place where tetanus and other infection can enter the baby. If you are using ties (sterilized white shoelaces do quite well), it is necessary to tie a *square knot* and to tie it as tightly as possible. When the cord is cut, there will be a tiny bit of blood, but after that there should be no bleeding or oozing from the cord. If there is, it should quickly be retied.

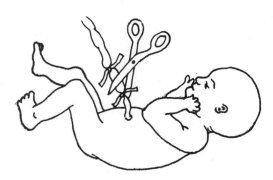

FIGURE 5-14. *Tying and cutting the cord.*

If you don't want to bother the baby right away, the cord can be cut long, and then retied two inches from the baby's skin and recut later (resterilize your scissors first).

Cut the cord with awareness. There are no nerve endings in the cord, so the baby doesn't feel anything, but it is a psychically significant event.

There is never any rush to cut the cord, unless it is wrapped tightly around the baby's neck and must be cut. You could even wait until the placenta is delivered, although the cord probably serves no purpose once it is white and limp. On the other hand, cutting the cord early is a shock to the baby, forcing him to depend on his lungs as the sole source of oxygen sooner than nature intended. Allowing the placental blood to flow into the baby also results in fewer third-stage complications for the mother and gives the baby greater iron stores. Some doctors may tell you that delayed cutting of the cord results in a high incidence of physiological jaundice, but the studies are inconclusive.

If the mother is Rh negative, the cord can be cut early to minimize the risk of blood incompatibility in the baby. If you are sure there aren't twins, then let the maternal end drain into a bowl to aid delivery of the placenta.

THIRD STAGE: DELIVERY OF THE PLACENTA

Once it is clear that the baby is breathing, attention should be placed on the mother, for the third stage is the most dangerous for you. Your vital signs should be good—good pulse, no pallor, clamminess or other signs of shock. The length of the cord should be pulled out of the vagina immediately after the birth, then someone should be watching it (with a flashlight if necessary) to see when it lengthens (one midwife I know puts an extra tie on it a few inches from the vagina as an indicator). Lengthening of the cord and a gush of blood are signs that the placenta has come away, and you should be helped to squat over a bowl to push the placenta out (gravity helps!).

The placenta usually separates within twenty or thirty minutes after the birth. You may feel a contraction—if so, you should be helped to squat. Nursing and nipple stimulation also cause the uterus to contract and can aid the placenta to be expelled.

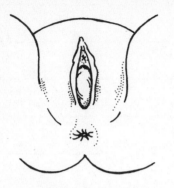

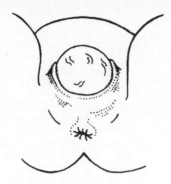

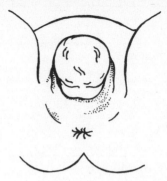

A. *The head appears at the vaginal opening.*

B. *Crowning.*

C. *Extension of the head as it emerges from under the pubic bone.*

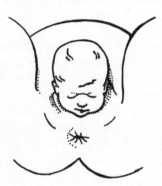

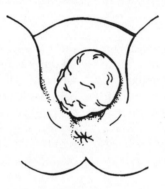

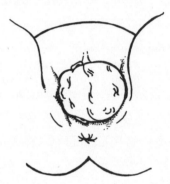

D. *Head drops back toward the rectum. Check to see if the cord is around the neck.*

E. *Restitution (turning back of the head).*

F. *Rotation of the head to allow birth of the shoulders.*

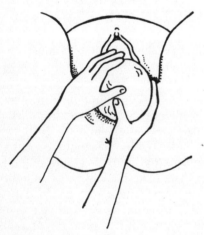

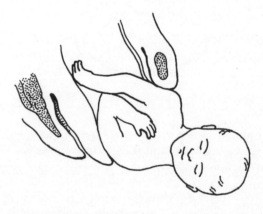

G. *The anterior (top) shoulder is born. Do not pull down on the head.*

H. *The top shoulder is usually delivered first, then the bottom one, and then the body slips out.*

FIGURE 5-13. *Another view of delivery.*

Don't pull on the cord. The uterus should not be massaged before the placenta has separated; that's one of the major causes of hemorrhage. Oxorn and Foote state this quite strongly:

> The most common cause of excessive bleeding is mismanagement of the third stage. The most frequent fault is to try to hasten delivery of the placenta before it has separated. Kneading or massaging the uterus roughly when it is not ready to contract may cause partial separation of the placenta and result in post-partum hemorrhage.[1]

If the placenta is in the bowl with membranes still attached to the mother, someone can gently twist the placenta around and around to dislodge the membranes. If you aren't paying attention and miss the separation of the placenta, you may run into difficulties (see Chapter 8).

BLEEDING

There will be a gush of blood when the placenta separates and more blood as it comes out, but after that the amount should quickly diminish. The uterus should be kept firm to seal off the blood vessels where the placenta has come away. Nursing and nipple stimulation help to firm the uterus, and someone should massage it every ten or fifteen minutes for the first hour. They should press their fingers in deeply on the sides of your uterus to encourage it to contract. However, avoid pushing down strongly from the top of the uterus, as the cervix may come down the vagina. Massaging up from the pubic bones along the ligaments connected to the uterus can also cause a contraction. Then when the uterus is palpated, it should feel round and hard, about the size of a grapefruit, and be situated below the belly button. If the uterus feels soft and boggy and you are bleeding, more massage and nipple stimulation should be done. (If bleeding continues, see Chapter 8.)

The total amount of blood loss should be estimated, including what is in the bowl (once it has separated from the amniotic fluid), and the amount on the sheets and pads. The total should be less than two cups, the hospital definition of hemorrhage.

If you continue to have a steady, slow trickle of blood and are soaking two sanitary pads in a half hour, you may have a slow-trickle hemorrhage, which is quite dangerous and needs to be controlled. Recheck the firmness of your uterus. Possible causes are retained fragments of the placenta, cervical lacerations or tears.

EXAMINING FOR TEARS

Examining for tears should be done with sterile gloves and close attention to sterile technique. Using a good light, your birth attendant will examine the external perineum, the clitoris, inner labia and urethra, and the pelvic floor muscles. If there are tears which require suturing in order to heal well, sterile gauze pads can usually be used to control the bleeding with pressure until the suturing can be done. There are three degrees of tearing, illustrated in Chapter 8.

If your birth attendant cannot do stitching, it is advisable to see a doctor within a couple of hours after the birth since many physicians feel the risk of infection is too great if suturing is done more than about five hours after an injury occurs.

EXAMINING THE PLACENTA

The placenta should be checked to see that it is complete. It is usually round and about one inch thick. The maternal side (Figure 5-15a) should have all the clumps (cotyledons) present. You can check by putting your hands underneath and lifting up the edges: the surface should all fit together smoothly. There may be a few "extra" pieces, which are clots, but there should be no pieces of placenta missing.

Occasionally a placenta has a separate lobe which may have remained in the uterus, so check the blood vessels on the baby's (shiny) side of the placenta (Figure 5-15b) to make sure that all the blood vessels end before the edge.

The membranes should also be checked. They should be complete so that if you pick them up they will form a sack with a hole at the top and the placenta at the bottom. They consist of two layers, the amnion and the chorion (Figure 5-15c).

Check the end of the cord. You should see three circles. These are the two arteries and the vein which form the cord (Figure 5-15d). If one is missing, you should have your baby checked by a pediatrician (this anomaly can be associated with certain birth defects).

If there are any questions about the placenta, take it with you to your doctor or clinic. If a piece has been retained, a curettage, or scraping of the uterus, may be done. Since it is often done under general anesthesia, don't eat or drink if you're having questions about the placenta.

BEING TOGETHER AS A FAMILY

As you can see, there's a lot to be aware of right after the birth. That's why most midwives bring an assistant,

---

[1]Harry Oxorn and William Foote, *Human Labor and Birth* (NY: Appleton-Century-Crofts, 1975), p. 120.

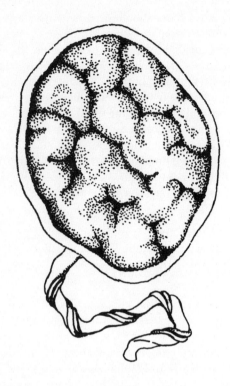

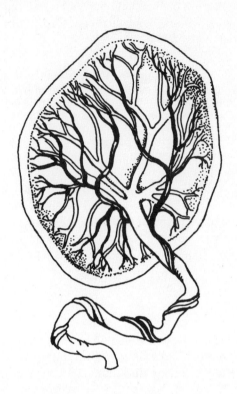

A. Maternal side of the placenta. Check to see that all the pieces (cotyledons) are there.

B. Baby's side of the placenta. All blood vessels should end before the edge.

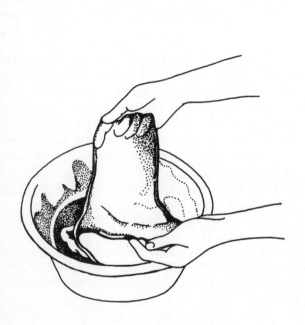

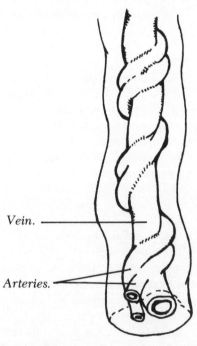

Vein.

Arteries.

C. Examining the membranes

D. Tying and cutting the cord. Check the end of the cord for two arteries and a vein.

FIGURE 5-15

so one can focus on the mother while the other focuses on the baby. You'll be able to hold your baby when he or she is first born, but you'll have to hand him or her to your partner while you squat to deliver the placenta.

Some fathers like to take off their shirts and hold the baby skin-to-skin, since babies are extremely sensitive to touch and smell. He may also wish to hold the baby in a warm bath at this point to relax the baby and release any tension that may have occurred in the birth process. Have enough water to cover the baby. The temperature should be about 99°F (it should feel warm when placed on the inside of the wrist or elbow). Have the bath near your bed so you can participate too. Place the baby gently in the water with two hands supporting his head and back.

Returning the baby to the weightless, warm state of the womb to ease the birth process is a procedure made famous by Dr. Frederick LeBoyer in *Birth Without Violence*. I feel there is an unfortunate tendency on the part of many people to ignore the thrust of what LeBoyer is saying and focus on this one act as the LeBoyer "technique." Certainly, anyone who has ever held a newborn in the water and felt the release in her body and seen her open up and start to play when only minutes old cannot feel that this is a fad or gimmick. But it is not necessary in every case. Holding and loving your baby may be just what she wants. LeBoyer's real message is simply awareness: awareness of this new being, and in particular of her needs to enter this new world gently, without the sensory overload of bright lights, loud sounds, rough touch and emotional insecurity. Even though Seth loved the bath, we didn't use it with Faith because she was so completely *there*, without tension or trauma. There are no fixed procedures. Read LeBoyer's book, and our description in Chapter 9, remember what birth feels like, and then see what your baby guides you to do.

Your baby will usually be awake and alert for a while right after the birth. A calm atmosphere in which you can be together and make eye contact helps the formation of family bonds. If you are going to use drops in the baby's eyes (required by law in many states), you might want to wait several hours, until the baby is sleepy, before putting them in. The drops are to protect the baby against blindness in case you have undetected gonorrhea, which babies can contract while coming down the birth canal. Silver nitrate has traditionally been used, but it burns the baby's eyes and can cause irritation for several days. Ilotycin and Argyrol are both effective and less traumatic to the eyes. If you are certain that you don't have gonorrhea (remembering that gonorrhea cultures are only about 80 percent effective in diagnosing the disease in women), and you decide not to use any drops, you should watch your baby closely and take it in immediately to have any eye discharge cultured if an infection develops. No one wants to risk blindness.

Your baby should be examined after birth by someone familiar with danger signs of the newborn (see Chapter 10). If you have any doubts or questions, get them checked out. There isn't any need to scrub the baby right away. The vernix, or cream cheese-like substance covering the baby, can be rubbed in, as it is excellent for the skin. Your baby should be dressed or wrapped enough to keep warm and avoid drafts, but the most important thing is that you touch, love and get to know one another.

CARE FOR THE MOTHER

Don't try to get up too soon, and have someone help you in the bathroom and in getting cleaned up. Drink some juice before trying to get up, and eat if you're hungry. When you first stand up, there will be a gush of blood that has accumulated in the vagina. Don't forget to urinate within about eight hours after the birth; your bladder may not be registering sensation yet, and you don't want it to get too full.

The main concerns for the mother post partum are excessive bleeding and infection. After the birth you should *not* be soaking two sanitary pads in a half hour, and the flow should diminish over the following days. If you develop a fever or your abdomen feels painful, see a doctor. You might want to take your temperature each morning for the first few days if you are concerned about infection; it should be under 100°F.

Once you are cleaned up, lie back, relax, eat, drink plenty of fluids, rest and sleep; and, above all, enjoy being with your baby and your partner.

NORMAL LABOR AND DELIVERY: SELF CHECK

These questions are oriented to the husband, who should have a firm understanding of labor and delivery, since he will be assuming an active role as coach. Use this as a learning process. Go back and look for answers to any questions you are not sure of.

1. What are the three ways labor can begin?
2. What should you do when the waters break?
3. What is effacement?
4. What is dilation?
   What causes it?
   How is it measured?
5. What does the bloody show during labor signify?
6. How often should the baby's heartbeat be listened to during labor? During pushing? What are the dangerous ranges?
7. What is transition? How will you know she is in it?
8. Why is it important that she not push in transition?

9. When should she start to push?
10. Once the head is visible at the vaginal opening, what should be done?
11. What is meant by crowning? How can you help her not to push then?
12. Once the head is out, what if the cord is around the neck?
13. Once the head is out, it rotates to the side. When are the shoulders born?
14. When and how would you suction the baby?
15. Reread the Apgar Scoring. What are you checking the newborn for?
16. How do you cut the cord? Why is sterile technique so important?
17. How can you tell if the placenta has come away from the uterus?
18. How can you help deliver the placenta?
19. How do you massage the uterus every fifteen minutes *after* the placenta is out? How should it feel?
20. How much blood loss constitutes hemorrhage?
21. What do you examine the placenta for? What would you do if it was incomplete?

22. Why are eyedrops placed in the baby's eyes? Do you or the birth attendant have the drops (what brand?)?

FOR FURTHER READING

A Guide to Midwifery: Heart and Hands by Elizabeth Davis. Highly recommended for its clear, comprehensive text and illustrations.

Emergency Childbirth by Dr. Gregory White. A guide for firemen, police and others who might find themselves at a birth. Good policy of "hands off, everything is normal," plus clear explanations of complications and emergency procedures.

Midwifery by Jean Hallum. A technical text that is short, clear and well-written.

Spiritual Midwifery by Ina May Gaskin. The section on management of normal labor in "Instructions to Midwives" is one of the best guides to labor and delivery.

ERIC SERGIO'S BIRTH—A PHOTO ESSAY

When Jenny was pregnant with Eric, she and Sergio and Posy, who had just turned four, were living in Michoacan, Mexico. Margaret, Wahhab and I went down for the time surrounding the birth. The entire labor took only three hours—so short that it took us days to believe it. Faith, our two and one-half year old couldn't stop repeating, "Jenny's baby came OUT!"

In the last three photographs, note Jenny squatting for the placenta; Margaret holding Eric Sergio in the bath (we had cut the cord long and held it out of the water); Mariposa holding her new baby brother. It was a really beautiful birth.

FIGURE 5-16

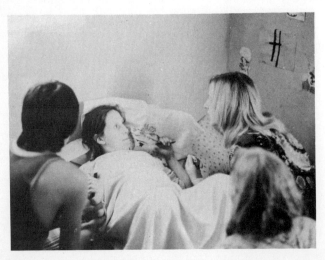

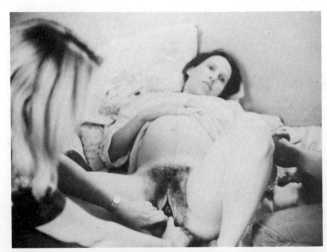

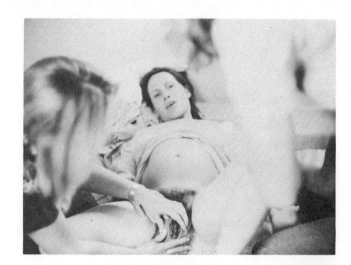
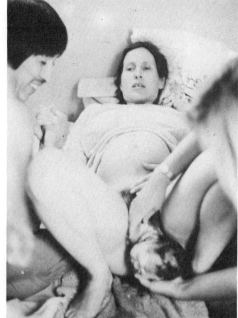
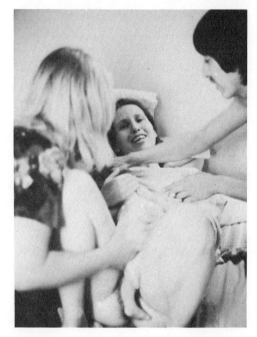
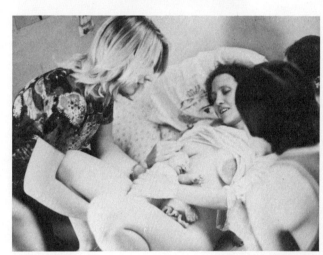
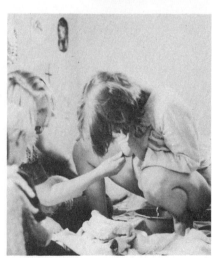
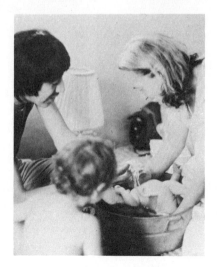
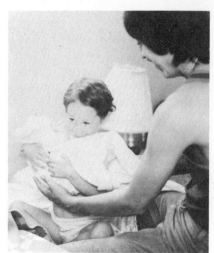

CHAPTER SIX

Tools for Handling Labor

CHILDBIRTH AND
CULTURAL CONDITIONING

Ideally, giving birth is a natural and joyful experience, a holy event in which the energies of creation and transformation can be shared by all who are present. Giving birth as a couple in your own home gives you the opportunity to fall in love all over again, both with the baby and with each other. Moreover, birth can be a transforming process, touching every aspect of your outlook on life.

Unfortunately, this experience is still not that of the majority of women in our culture. Instead, they live through a largely self-fulfilling prophecy of birth as a painful, terrifying ordeal, and/or as a medical, drugged process over which they have no control.[1] Birth is powerfully influenced by our attitudes and ideas. The images we have of giving birth, our expectations, conditioning and body image, determine not only how we react, but the length of labor, its progress, and how we feel afterwards. Until I understood the range of factors operative in labor and delivery, I used to wonder how birth in the West and the typical four-hour labors in some pre-medicalized cultures (even for first babies)

could involve the same female body and physiological function!

Our culture still carries much of the idea that childbirth is a fearful and painful experience. It is both exciting and enlightening when these concepts suddenly fall away in the light of new revelation. This happened to Dr. Grantly Dick-Read early in this century when he offered chloroform to a woman in labor, who declined and said somewhat guiltily afterwards, "But it isn't *supposed* to hurt, is it?" Read's contemplation of this woman led him to develop "natural childbirth." A similar experience occurred to Dr. Fernand Lamaze thirty years later, when he visited Russia and observed women giving birth with smiles on their faces. And a similar thing happened to me when I was contemplating having a baby, wondering how anyone as cowardly as I could ever survive the process, and discovered through the various methods of preparation that having a baby could be an exciting, joyful experience. Perhaps our children will grow up familiar with birth and knowing it to be a positive, fulfilling process, but for most of us that discovery, and a corresponding effort of deconditioning, must occur when we become pregnant or are contemplating having a child.

ABOUT PAIN

Although we tend to assume that what hurts, hurts, psychologists have discovered that there are many factors that influence our experience of pain. Those factors influencing birth are summarized in the accompanying list.

---

[1] Studies have estimated that only 10 percent of the pregnant couples in this country attend prepared childbirth classes that can give them the tools to enjoy an aware birth. And yet women who have been anesthetized have the subconscious realization that birth is something more; this may be expressed as vague dissatisfaction, or the feeling that they have missed something or have had a terrible experience. For a detailed comparison of the psychological impact of birth on prepared and unprepared mothers, see Deborah Tanzer's *Why Natural Childbirth? A Psychologist's Report on Benefits to Mothers, Fathers, and Babies* (New York: Schocken, 1976).

FACTORS IN LABOR WHICH AFFECT THE EXPERIENCE OF PAIN

Increase

Hunger
Tiredness
Focus on pain
Worry, uncertainty
Tension
Fear of unknown
Loneliness
Waiting for the pain
Feeling helpless

Decrease

Satisfaction
Being rested
Focus on others and environment
Confidence
Relaxation
Knowledge
Company of partner and friends
Focus on the present
Being self-determined and active

Hunger is best dealt with by eating light foods during early labor and drinking juices to keep up your blood sugar level. (The hospital procedure of refusing food and drink to women in labor in case general anesthesia is required then necessitates the use of routine IV drips).

Tiredness can be prevented by resting your last month of pregnancy, sleeping through early labor if it is night, and relaxing fully between contractions.

Focus on the pain intensifies it. Everyone is familiar with how overwhelming a toothache or headache can be, until a special friend says, "Let's go to the movies." After the movie, the toothache is still there—and indeed, it was present all the time—but while your attention was directed externally it didn't register in your consciousness. Staying focused on your surroundings, your partner and the purpose of labor are invaluable tools in helping you deal successfully with contractions.

Worry and uncertainty are handled by preparation: taking classes, knowing what to expect, and being able to interpret what is happening with your body. A good coach can help immensely in maintaining confidence.

Tension is probably the major cause of pain in labor. A baby is born through contraction of the uterine muscle, the strongest muscle in the human body. If the rest of your body is relaxed, your uterus can do its work effectively, without the pain or exhaustion of muscular tension in your abdomen, legs or shoulders. Relaxation, aided by the touch, encouragement and attention of those who love you, is the key to a comfortable and joyous labor.

Waiting for the pain is self-fulfilling because it causes tension, which actually creates pain. It can cause all your past experiences of pain to become jumbled together and be carried into the present, along with all the fears of the future. Experiencing each contraction and each rest period as each one comes solves this problem, for the experience in a given moment is never so intense that it cannot be accepted. Staying in the here-and-now is one of your best tools.

In addition to these factors, our experience of pain is influenced by our attitude towards it. If we can simply recognize pain for what it is, a sensation our body is registering to inform us of our situation, and meet it calmly and dispassionately, our body can accept the message we send back: "Thank you. I know what's happening. I don't need any further signals right now."

METHODS OF PREPARED CHILDBIRTH

The Read Method, which popularized the term *natural childbirth*, was based on Dr. Grantly Dick-Read's formulation in the 1920s of the fear-tension-pain triangle: fear of the unknown causes tension, which results in pain, which causes fear of more pain, etc. He found that breaking this vicious cycle by replacing fear with knowledge about birth and by replacing tension with relaxation resulted in a great reduction in the pain experienced by a laboring woman.

In America the *Read Method* has been almost entirely supplanted by the *Lamaze Method*, also termed *Psychoprophylaxis*, or using the mind to prevent pain. This was developed by Dr. Fernand Lamaze around 1950, based on the Pavlovian system which he discovered being used in Russia. The method emphasizes deconditioning the connection between pain and contractions that a woman has learned and reconditioning her to respond with certain breathing patterns, to focus her vision on a single point, and to respond to the verbal commands of her coach. Rapid, panting breathing is used during strong contractions, although the recommended breathing has slowed down considerably over the years.

Dr. Robert Bradley developed the *Bradley Method*, or *husband-coached childbirth*, as a method of "true natural childbirth." It uses only slow breathing, the kind of breathing that he states all mammals with sweat glands use in giving birth. Bradley was the originator of training the husband as coach and having him present in the delivery room as an integral part of the birthing team, and he emphasizes that almost all Bradley- trained couples go through birth without any anesthesia at all.

The psycho-sexual method of prepared childbirth, developed by Sheila Kitzinger in England, involves recognizing that birth is an integral part of a couple's psychological and sexual lives and working with these factors as well as with breathing and relaxation. She emphasizes being willing to feel sensation and to open to the birthing experience rather than trying for a "painless" birth.

In the United States today, most prepared childbirth classes are Lamaze or modified Lamaze, with Bradley and holistic classes such as informed birth and parenting being offered. Because of the immense individual variation between teachers, with many combining techniques from various sources, you should talk with teachers to see what they actually teach rather than searching for a "method."

PREPARATION AND PAIN

It is my personal feeling that women do better learning to say *yes* to sensation and opening to birth, which is extremely intense and may even be uncomfortable/painful at times, rather than trying for a painless childbirth.

Lamaze called his method *accouchement sans douleur,* or "childbirth without pain." When my first labor really hurt and I didn't look like the smiling woman I had seen in the movie in our Lamaze class, I felt I had failed, that I must be doing something wrong. This led me to become a childbirth educator to get to the bottom of the mystery of whether childbirth could really be painless. It is my conclusion from working with couples trained in the current Lamaze tradition, and noting the large percentage who use anesthesia, that the emphasis on painless childbirth (and on not feeling guilty about using anesthesia if you do feel pain) can be a misleading one.

I have, in fact, seen two women give birth completely without pain or discomfort. Both were having their second baby and although both had been bothered by "Braxton-Hicks" contractions, neither ever felt labor contractions, even through transition. These women have certainly been the exception, however. What I can say from my experience in having two children and teaching hundreds of couples is that, for most women, birth is an incredibly intense experience, and although a contraction need not be interpreted as painful, it is, in Ina May Gaskin's words, "an interesting sensation requiring all your attention!" Giving birth is usually one of the most intense experiences of your entire life.

When you prepare for your birth and approach it with confidence, the amount of pain and discomfort which you will experience during labor and birth will be greatly decreased. You will have the confidence and the tools to handle whatever your labor may bring you and to experience it as a joyous event.

ATTENDING CLASSES

Even if you have a good theoretical grasp of breathing and relaxation, attending classes will provide you with an opportunity for regular practice, and can get your partner more immediately involved with the pregnancy and birth. Classes also provide a chance to get to know other pregnant couples, and can give you a lot better understanding of birth through slides, films and other visual aids.

See "Resources in Your Community" on p. 52 for how to find homebirth or prepared-childbirth classes.

EMOTIONAL PREPARATION

Fear of pain, fear of failure, or unresolved emotions from past births, miscarriages or abortions can negatively influence your feelings and decisions so your present birth is also less than ideal. Pregnancy is a good time for clearing out trapped emotions from such past experiences. The exercises in *Pregnant Feelings, Transformation Through Birth* and *Silent Knife* can provide valuable tools for approaching this birth with as much clarity as possible (see references at the end of this chapter).

RELAXATION: THE KEY TO LABOR

The key to "staying on top of" contractions is *relaxation.* Rather than breathing faster or trying forty-seven different positions to get comfortable (which may be impossible), *relax more.* Be there, in the present moment; center your attention in the breath and keep telling your body to release. And enjoy it! Although labor is hard work and can be extremely intense, you're not going to be pregnant very much longer, and you're not going to be experiencing labor and birth for very long (or probably very many times, either), so savor it all—it involves a whole set of new sensations and emotions.

Pain is increased by tension in the body. Keeping any set of muscles contracted for the duration of labor is going to be very uncomfortable. Your uterus relaxes in between contractions, and the rest of your body should be relaxed all the time. Pain is also caused by resisting (which results in more tension and pain) rather than experiencing the sensation without the mental interpretation that it has to be painful. What we are aiming for is a completely relaxed body in which the contracting uterus is allowed to do its work of opening the cervix while you conserve your energy.

Relaxation is not a passive process. It is a self-directed interaction between your body and mind. How can you stay relaxed during labor? One of your main tools is intention: you are going to sit or lie there, completely relaxed, while strong uterine sensations recur from time to time, and tell your body and your various groups of muscles (especially those in your shoulders and lower belly) to release, relax and stay relaxed.

Practice and repetition are helpful, for they teach the body new response patterns, which then become automatic (like learning how to type). By practicing breathing and relaxation exercises regularly, your body can learn to greet strong sensation with relaxation and the breath, rather than with tension, recoiling and holding the breath, as we usually do. This relearning will come to your aid in all stressful situations, from experiencing emotional turmoil to going to the dentist.

BREATHING: TO KEEP YOU RELAXED

Your breath is intimately connected with all your physical and emotional states. It not only reflects them, it also can produce them; professional actors often use the breath in this way to produce emotions on stage.

Use the breath as a tool. Keep centered in it; that is, place your attention on your breathing, and feel as if you are floating in the middle of the breath. In addition, *keep it as slow as possible.* Many people who have been trained in the Lamaze Method (which uses shallow, panting breathing for strong contractions) don't really believe it is possible to maintain slow breathing throughout labor, but the Bradley Method teaches only slow breathing, and it really does work! With only slow breathing, you end up much more relaxed, are more in touch with your body, don't run the risk of hyperventilating, and enjoy labor more because you aren't fluttering around the ceiling doing rapid breathing.

BREATHING BETWEEN CONTRACTIONS

Let your breathing be relaxed throughout labor. In between contractions, the breath can actually dispel tension and help you relax. Use each outbreath to relax a little more deeply. Let the breath fill your entire body, surrounding and relaxing each muscle; wherever you feel tension, use the outbreath to send it away.

BREATHING DURING CONTRACTIONS

Intentionally doing slow breathing during contractions provides a focal point for your concentration, keeping you centered and calm through each contraction as it builds and subsides. The breathing helps you stay relaxed, and when you are relaxed, your breath flows slowly and rhythmically (another plus for slow breathing). Breathe with deep, slow breaths, raising your belly up off your uterus (diaphragmatic or "sleep" breathing.) Actually moving your belly during contractions assures that your breaths are deep and keeps the muscles in your lower belly from becoming tense and painful during contractions (see photos).

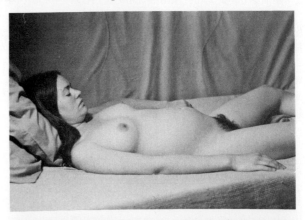

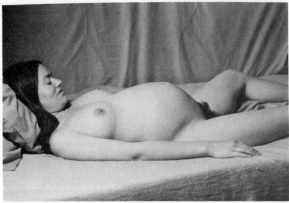

FIGURES 6-1, 6-2. *Breathing is deep and full, so your belly raises up off your uterus when you inhale.*

The cleansing breath is a really deep sigh at the beginning and end of each contraction, signaling to those around you that you are having a contraction, and signaling yourself that it is time to concentrate again. The cleansing breaths serve as punctuation marks for your experience. You greet each contraction with relaxation and a deep breath and then say goodbye to it at the end (you'll never see that one again!), releasing any tension that may have crept in.

It's a good idea to relax completely for a few seconds after the final cleansing breath and feel throughout your entire body, releasing any tension which may have

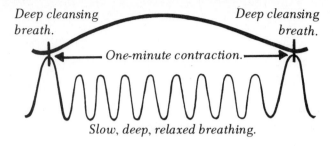

Deep cleansing breath.

One-minute contraction.

Deep cleansing breath.

Slow, deep, relaxed breathing.

FIGURE 6-3. *Slow, deep relaxed breathing through a contraction.*

accumulated. Then turn to your coach, give each other feedback on what worked, what you felt, what you need, and so forth. Figure 6-3 shows how breathing during labor might be visualized.

ENERGY AND ATTITUDE

At a birth, you, the laboring woman, are the channel for the Life Force, the energy of creation and transformation. As such, you need to be completely open to the birth process. There is no right or wrong way to "behave" in labor—you can breathe or bellow, doing what you need to do to maintain equilibrium at the same time that you surrender to the power of birth. It's not unlike surfing or skiing.

If you're like a huge sponge, soaking up all the energy from your partner, midwife and friends, things are likely to get constipated. If you can put out energy, more can flow through you. For example, hug and kiss with your husband, really giving to him and letting him share in the powerful energies coursing through you. Saying "I love you" to your partner or friends is saying it to your baby and can really help you to open up. Be positive in all that you say. If you're finding it difficult to stay on top (if some of the old "tapes" that still clutter our minds are vying for attention), make positive statements about what you are trying to do, like "I'm opening up," or "I'm relaxing more and more." If you are having difficulties or need something, ask your attendants for it. If you are having some doubt or fear, verbalize it. You may get the information or reassurance you need, or just stating it may help. Unconscious or repressed fears directly influence your body and your labor. *Pregnant Feelings* discusses working with the energy of birth in great detail.

INTERACTING WITH YOUR PARTNER

A husband and wife form a single energy unit during a birth. If there is any negativity or lack of acceptance between you, try to get it handled before the birth, other-

wise you may have to work it out during labor, which is not the only thing you will have on your minds at that time! Give to each other, nurture each other, all during pregnancy and especially during the birth. Be sensitive to each other's needs and be gateful for the other's attention and affection.

TOOLS FOR GOOD LABOR SUPPORT

Your partner will probably be your primary support, and he plays an invaluable role in helping you stay relaxed and enjoy your labor. But other friends can also fulfill that function for the single mother or can relieve your partner during labor. Here are some of the tools your support people can use.

AFFIRMATION

Please don't be fooled by the word "coach" into thinking that this is the place for athletic competition. Your job is to help and encourage your wife to deal with the process of labor as best she can. There is no right or wrong way for her to do this, and there is no ideal against which she is being measured or graded. You will usually be much more helpful to her by giving her praise than by criticizing her. Tell her that she's just had a good strong contraction and that she's doing fine. If she got tense during that contraction, encourage her verbally and with touch to relax more while she has the next one. Be accepting, but don't forget that you have a responsibility to actively help her with her relaxation and her labor.

COMMUNICATION

After a contraction, see if she likes what you did. During early labor you usually have at least five minutes between contractions, plenty of time for discussion and for working together to greet each succeeding contraction with more relaxation than the last.

During active labor or transition, however, she may need to conserve her strength and may not feel like talking. So know that if she brushes your hand away, it's a way of saying that it no longer feels good and is not a rejection of your efforts. Realize too that as labor progresses, what feels good or what is needed changes, and be as receptive to her needs as you can. Sometimes in transition *nothing* feels good, and she may start giving you contradictory messages or not knowing what she wants. Recognize that this is one of the symptoms of transition, and does not reflect on the value of your presence with her. Remind her that the strong contractions are opening her cervix so the baby can be born.

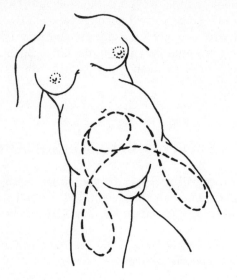

FIGURE 6-4a. *Light massage by partner.*

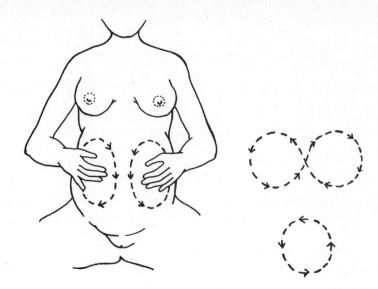

FIGURE 6-4b. *Self circles.*

BEING HERE-AND-NOW

In each present moment, either the uterus is contracting (and anyone can bear 60 seconds of intense sensation), or the body is at rest. By keeping her focused on the present moment rather than "how long it's been" or "how much longer it's going to be," you help her to accept and deal with what she's actually feeling. If she is losing her concentration, orient her to the objects in the room, point to something outside the window, have her look at the people who are there, ask her to describe what she is actually feeling. And then use direct, eye-to-eye contact during the following contractions.

NON-VERBAL COMMUNICATION

You really know her body and can see where she is tense. Strengthening your non-verbal communication through touch relaxation (described here), you can help her body directly by encouraging tense areas to release towards your hand.

MASSAGE

A light, circular massage of her belly and upper legs often feels good during contractions and helps keep the legs from pulling in. Rub gently but definitely, using the entire hand, always keeping it in contact with the body to eliminate her uncertainty about where it's going to come down next (Figure 6-4a). She can also lightly massage herself during contractions (Figure 6-4b).

She may experience a lot of lower-back pain as the baby descends lower in the birth canal and presses against the sacrum. It can be even more intense if the back of the baby's head is pressing against her backbone (back labor). You can help by using firm, strong, continuous counterpressure during a contraction on both sides of the spine in the area of the sacrum. Pushing up on the ischial tuberosities (the sit bones) can also help. Again, use strong, continuous counterpressure during the contraction.

Grasping the inner thigh or the lower belly sometimes feels good and helps her to release, and stimulating the nipples can help the uterus to contract and help labor along (Figure 6-5).

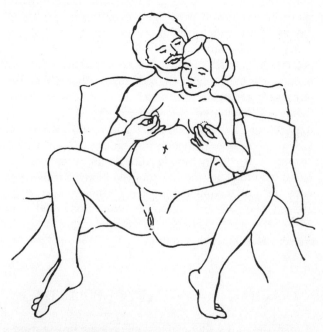

FIGURE 6-5. *Nipple stimulation produces oxytocin, which stimulates labor.*

WORKING WITH INTENSE CONTRACTIONS

Encourage her to stay with the slow breathing. During the strongest contractions, help her keep on top by establishing eye-to-eye contact and breathing with her during the contraction, emphasizing the outbreath. If she loses her breathing rhythm or feels she can't go on, you may need to be very firm and directive, getting her complete attention and insisting that she breathe with you during the contraction. She will be much more comfortable if you actively work with her during these strongest contractions and keep her attention. Don't let her get lost in a contraction or labor. Establish in advance that you will blow out together and then breathe together with direct eye contact. It really does work. If she loses the breathing during a contraction, have her blow out, and then reestablish the rhythm with her.

After the contraction, help her smooth her body out and breathe directly with her during the next one. Unless you are using the Lamaze rapid breathing, keep her breath slow and deep.

Help her to relax, both verbally and through your touch and manner. Placing a hand on her lower belly early in labor, and making sure that her breathing is moving all those muscles, will also help prevent tension.

Probably at no other time in marriage do you express your love so directly, unselfishly and effectively as during labor. Your care, direct attention and love provide her with immense support.

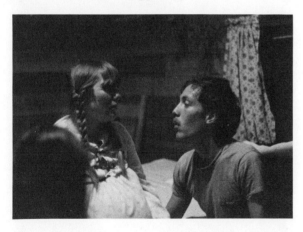

FIGURE 6-6. *Use eye contact and breathe with her during strong contractions.*

POSITIONS FOR LABOR

Being vertical is the best position for labor in terms of the strength and frequency of contractions and how fast your cervix dilates. Studies done in a hospital in Spain found that the effectiveness of contractions in dilating the cervix was doubled in the standing position and that mothers found this position much less uncomfortable

---

HAND REFLEXOLOGY AND LABOR

In one edition of the "Informed Homebirth Newsletter" we reviewed the book *Hand Reflexology: The Key to Perfect Health* by Mildred Carter, and got very positive responses from women who tried grasping combs during labor.

Carter holds that the reason women have traditionally clutched bedposts, hands of attendants, etc., is that those spots in the hand directly relate to the uterus, and that pressure on the balls of the hand and on the mid-finger tips facilitates smooth, rapid and relatively painless functioning of the uterus. Carter suggests holding two strong combs so that they press on the pressure points of each hand, squeezing tightly during contractions and relaxing between them.

The births I have attended where the women have used the combs have gone very rapidly, and the women felt the combs helped them to relax (Figure 6-7). It's a good tool to try, especially if you have a sluggish labor.

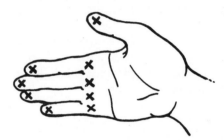

FIGURE 6-7. *Grasping on comb presses on acupressure points.*

---

and painful than lying on their backs.[2] In the study, they alternated women standing and lying on their backs at half-hour intervals. The mean length of labor in their study group of primigravidas was less than four hours, and none required analgesia.

Another study in the United States found that propping women up at a 30° angle for labor and delivery resulted in a greater regularity and frequency of uterine contractions and a shorter first and second stage than among the control group.[3]

Women in all cultures other than those practicing Western obstetrics adapt standing, kneeling and squatting postures for labor and delivery. Many rural Mexican women in Guerrero, for example, hang a rope from

---

[2] Peter M. Dunn, "Obstetric Delivery Today, For Better or for Worse?" *The Lancet*, April 10, 1976, p. 793.

[3] Yuen Chou Liu, "Effects of an Upright Position During Labor," *American Journal of Nursing*, December 1974, pp. 2202–05.

the ceiling which they hold onto in a kneeling position, with the buttocks resting on the heels. As Dr. Roberto Caldeyro-Barcia, president of the International Federation of Gynecologists and Obstetricians, stated, "Except for being hanged by the feet, the supine position (flat on the back) is the worst conceivable position for labor and delivery."[4] It can cause compression of the maternal blood vessels supplying the uterus and result in maternal hypotension and fetal distress. It also leads to a loss of gravity, less efficient uterine contractions, longer labor and greater discomfort. And it decreases the ability of the pelvis to open and makes the birth canal narrower.[5]

Sit or lie down when you are feeling tired or when you need to relax, but the more you are able to be vertical, the better your labor should progress. When you lie down, lie on your left side (the best for your circulation), or propped up in the contour position with lots of pillows.

Squatting is your best aid for increasing contractions, speeding up progress or helping the baby down the birth canal. It's a difficult position for those of us who don't squat while we work (unlike women in many other cultures), so have your friends support you or hold onto a bed or the back of a chair, and sit back between contractions.

Films from France and Brazil show urban women birthing in a supported squatting position without perineal support, since pressure is equally distributed all around the vaginal opening.

PRACTICING RELAXATION

Relaxing is often thought of as being passive, but in labor it is something you have to do actively. No one can relax for you. Your coach will help greatly, but it is you who must focus your attention and intention and release your muscles, just as, for example, you consciously release in difficult yoga postures. First, read through the following section with your coach. Then, to practice, lie in a comfortable position, with enough pillows to support your head and knees. Uncross your feet and let your arms lie comfortably by your side. Make sure the room is warm and the lighting comfortable. Then practice the exercises, having your coach read them to you. The entire series of exercises is summarized at the end of the chapter.

---

[4]In *Family Practicioner News*, 5:11, 1975.

[5]X-ray studies have shown that the cross sectional surface area of the birth canal may increase by as much as 30 percent when a woman changes from the dorsal to the squatting position. Dunn, *op. cit.*, pp. 792–93.

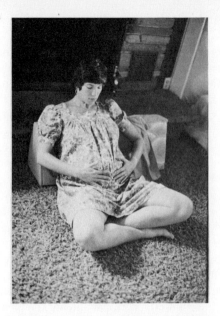

FIGURE 6-8. *Sitting cross-legged, doing light massage.*

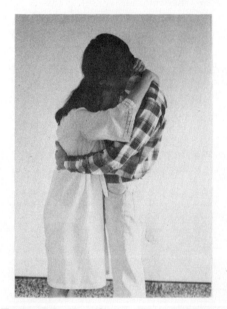

FIGURE 6-9. *Standing with your partner.*

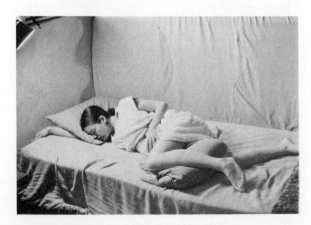

FIGURE 6-10. *Side relaxation position.*

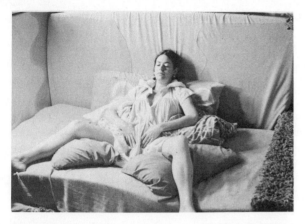

FIGURE 6-11. *Contour position, with lots of pillows.*

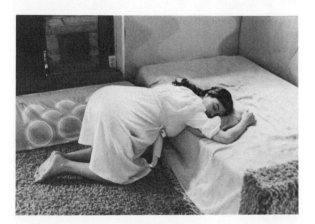

FIGURE 6-12. *Hands and knees—especially comfortable if supported by a bed or low table with pillows. Good for back labor.*

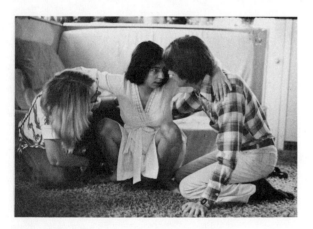

FIGURE 6-13. *Squatting with support.*

CALMING THE MIND

Sometimes your mind is racing and your emotions have you tied in knots. This may be true when you can't sleep, and it may be true in early labor when the excite-

ment and adrenaline rush of "This is it! Can I do it? Is everything together? What about the . . ." can make early labor much more strenuous than it need be.

A good method of calming the mind is centering in the breath. If done for twenty minutes daily until your baby is born, it can help you meet labor (or any other situation) with more calm and clarity.

CENTERING IN THE BREATH

Sit in a relaxed posture with the spine vertical. An upright chair is fine, or you can sit on pillows with your legs crossed. Facing a blank wall or a plain rug, leave your eyes and your mouth relaxed. Rest your hands, palms upward, on your thighs.

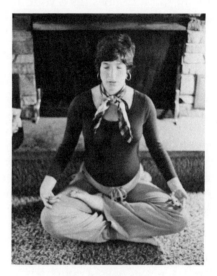

FIGURE 6-14.

Now focus your attention on your breath. Don't try to change your breathing; simply watch the natural flow of the breath in and out of the body. Don't try to shut other things out of your consciousness; just choose to have your focal point be the breath.

When you notice your attention drifting, simply return it to the breath. There is no need to make any special effort to suspend thoughts, although with regular practice thoughts will gradually begin to fall away.

This exercise is best practiced at a regular time and place. Doing some stretching exercises and then washing the hands and face with cold water before starting will also help keep the body and mind from complaining.

CENTERING IN LABOR

CLARITY Focus your mind by placing your attention in your body. Watch your breathing. Every emotion has a characteristic holding or altering of the breath pattern. Allow the breath to be full and deep, so that your body, your emotions, and your mind all release. Remain centered in the breath and let your thoughts fall away.

RELEASING THE BODY.   The breath is also the best tool for releasing the body.

RELEASE Let your breath deepen, so you are breathing all the way down into your belly. Let your body feel heavy, as if it were sinking into foam rubber or into warm sand at the beach. Breathe with your diaphragm, as you do during sleep.

As your breathing becomes slower, use each breath to release more fully. On the outbreath, let go of any holding or tension that may be in your body. Feel the breath flowing all the way down your backbone so there is a connection between your tailbone and the top of your head. Let the breath surround your baby and go all the way into your vagina and anus, making sure they are both released.

WHOLE BODY RELAXATION Now use your attention to travel throughout your body, releasing on the outbreath any tension you may find. Start with your face and eyes, cheeks and jaws. Travel down through the neck and shoulders, then the chest and belly, paying special attention to the muscles of the lower belly and upper legs. If you find any places of chronic tension which don't release with the breath, imagine the area to be warm, and imagine your outbreath flowing through it. (Also note these chronic places to work on with your partner).

This state of complete relaxation is one which you should know intimately, and be able to return to at will. Practice when you can't sleep, when you're sitting in the dentist's office (you don't have to be lying down!), or the next time you have too much to do and are feeling frazzled. Complete release is the key to comfort in labor.

WORKING WITH YOUR PARTNER

Being told "Relax your shoulders" is nowhere near as effective as feeling a loving, relaxing touch. The body responds on a body level, through non-verbal communication, the language of touch. Your partner knows your body intimately, and by working together now, touching and *communicating* about what helps you to release, you can work together as a loving and effective team during labor.

Massage.

Get into full-body massage with some of the body oils or lotions that make you feel good. Being pregnant is an especially good time to be in touch with each other and to feel the baby both physically and psychically. And give your partner massages and backrubs too—it not only makes him feel good, but lets you experience what feedback you would like from him so you can be more responsive when he's working with you in labor.

Touch.

Build up a pattern within your body of releasing to your partner's touch.

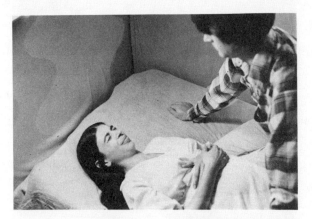

FIGURE 6-15. *Tense the muscles of your forehead.*

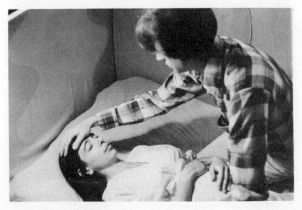

FIGURE 6-16. *Now release to his touch.*

TOUCH RELAXATION Partner: Tell her to contract her forehead. Then touch it with your whole hand, not massaging, but just lifting off the tension. Actually imagine energy flowing into your hand and out through you. Take your hand off, tell her to contract another set of muscles. Place your hand on the tension and encourage her to release to your touch. Continue, using other parts of the body, starting at the top of her head and working down. Take your hand off between contractions so you are only touching her when you want her to release. Make sure she releases fully to your touch, and use a touch which encourages release.

Mother: release to his touch, allowing tension to flow into his hand. By practicing this regularly, you will build up an association of releasing to the touch. Then in labor, when someone touches you, your body will unconsciously release toward the touch. You can also practice this while having a pelvic exam, and it will be much more comfortable. For a more detailed description of touch relaxation and other excellent exercises for body awareness and relaxation, see *The Experience of Childbirth* by Sheila Kitzinger.

Sharing Energy.

Some evenings you can set aside a time to share energy together. Lying in bed naked together, begin by touching one another, hugging and kissing. Then try to feel the totality of each other's bodies, inside and out, and feel the energy flowing between you. Allow the energy to flow, and consciously release any blocks you feel. Feel the presence of the baby, and allow energy to flow among the three of you. Welcome the baby, telling her you are looking forward to her joining you in the exciting world of sights, smells and touch.

It is important in this sharing not to be goal-directed, not to be trying to turn each other on or to reach any particular state, but simply to be sharing what is, in a loving and friendly way. Don't be afraid to verbalize any feelings. For a more detailed discussion of sexuality during pregnancy, see *Pregnant Feelings*.

PRACTICING CONTRACTIONS

When you are actually in labor there will be time between contractions for you to relax fully, talking with each other if it is early labor, being massaged, or doing whatever helps you to release. During contractions, you will be doing the slow, deep breathing which can help keep you centered. It can also be helpful to tell your body, "Okay, this really strong sensation is going on, but I'm staying really released and open." Direct your attention to any problem areas and tell them to release. The shoulders, the lower belly, and the legs are areas that may require special help.

RELAXATION CHECK Partner: Check her relaxed state (from the previous exercises) by picking up an arm or a leg with both hands, lifting it firmly and gently. Encourage her to let the limb be heavy, so she isn't helping you lift it. Be trustworthy! Help her feel that you won't drop it. As you put it down, help the shoulder and hip joints to release and widen by gently running your hands down the extremity and out the tips of the fingers or toes. When you put the arm or leg down, it should feel more released than the other side. Then do the other side, to help her feel symmetrical again.

PRACTICE CONTRACTION Signal to her, "Contraction begins." She should take a deep cleansing breath. Then she should do slow, deep, relaxed breathing throughout the "contraction." She should breathe from the diaphragm, so her belly raises up off the uterus on the inbreath. Placing your hand there can help her to feel if she is moving those muscles, which otherwise tend to become contracted along with the uterus. Maintain the contraction for about a minute, and then say, "Contraction ends." She will give another deep cleansing breath. After she releases completely for a few seconds, talk about what has just occurred and whether there are ways to improve the next contraction experience.

For another variation, act as her uterus, simulating a contraction by squeezing the inside of her thigh. Start by squeezing gently (you won't need to tell her "Contraction begins," as she'll feel it). Build up to a fairly tight squeeze. Encourage her to maintain the slow breathing, and then release slowly. Remember, your purpose is to encourage her to greet the sensation with the breath and stay relaxed throughout. Wait a few minutes and do another one.

WHAT ABOUT RAPID BREATHING?

During active labor, your contractions will be stronger and it will require more concentration to maintain the slow breathing. This slow relaxed breathing will help with all your contractions, keeping your body relaxed and your mind focussed. It is much easier on your throat and expends less energy than shallow, rapid breathing. It also assures that you don't hyperventilate and that your baby receives adequate oxygen.

However, if you are accustomed to rapid breathing in labor, or find that on the very heaviest contractions it helps you to breathe more rapidly, then make the breath *light and shallow,* centered in the mouth. Avoid rapid chest breathing, which can lead to hyperventilation, a condition that makes you feel light-headed, makes your hands and feet start to feel numb and go into claw position, and is not good for your baby. If you feel any of these symptoms, cup your hands over your mouth and nose and rebreathe your own air—and then change your breathing!

RECLAIMING SECOND STAGE

When Seth was born, my Lamaze training and my birth attendants had me push so hard that, even though I only pushed seven or eight times, and panted for the crowning, I tore quite badly and was stiff across the shoulders the next day. Convinced that there had to be a better way, I was excited to find an entirely different approach to pushing in Sheila Kitzinger's *The Experience of Childbirth.* With Faith, I didn't push at all, and was amazed to find myself opening up, allowing her to be born with no straining. I also felt this caused Faith to have a much more comfortable journey, and I wanted to share this approach to second stage.

If you find yourself in agreement with the approach described here, show this section to your birth attendant so she will understand what you are trying to do and will not be working at cross purposes with you. You may find more restrictions from hospital staff who still think you have to strain, but "responsive pushing" is gradually gaining acceptance in this country.

Second stage is said to begin once your cervix is fully dilated and ends when your baby is born. Once your cervix is fully dilated, the nature of your contractions will change. They will feel different than they did in transition, and they will be further apart (perhaps every three minutes). As the baby's head descends and pushes against your rectum, you will feel as if you need to have a bowel movement or your breath will involuntarily catch during the peak of a contraction. You are starting to feel the urge to push.

Much of the teaching in prepared-childbirth classes and many films of prepared couples giving birth, even at home, show an intensely athletic second stage. The woman is clutching her legs (if there are no stirrups, she can often be seen at home imitating the stirrup position, which is ridiculous). Her attendants are acting like cheerleaders, and the doctor is urging her to "Keep pushing! Keep the baby down! Don't let it slide back an inch," which sounds to me as if he's ready to catch the baby like a football and run with it! This approach has the woman holding her breath and pushing for the duration of every contraction from the time she is fully dilated until the head crowns (which can range anywhere from a few contractions in a multipara to two or three hours in a first birth).

I advocate the revolutionary view that you feel each contraction and add your own pushing efforts only when a specific contraction demands it (i.e. takes you with it). This allows you to fully feel the baby descend, and to give birth calmly without becoming exhausted.

Despite our cultural images to the contrary, there is no need for haste in the second stage. Even prolonged second stages, three hours and longer, show no greater incidence of hemorrhage, infection or distress in the baby (see Cohen's study under "Complications of Second Stage" in Chapter 8). As long as your baby's heartbeat is good (it should be checked every ten minutes in second stage), there is no need either to bring the head down quickly or to get it out as rapidly as possible.

But everyone is eager to see the baby, and no one wants second stage to go on longer than necessary. Does strenuous, athletic pushing really help to get the baby out any better or faster? The studies of Constance Beynon[6] found that when 100 normal primigravidas with vertex presentations were allowed to follow their own inclinations, when "pushing" was not mentioned by the women's birth attendants and they were not hurried at all, 83 of the women delivered completely spontaneously, without strain. Only two of these had second stages lasting over two hours, with the average being one hour and 3 minutes. Fifteen of these babies weighed over 8 pounds, three over 9 pounds, and one weighed 10 lbs. 9 oz.! Seventeen cases were given exhortation in pushing, usually after two hours (but Beynon states that some of these may not really have required it then). Of these, only six ended in forceps delivery—about half the rate of the control group. And only 39 of the 100 required episiotomies or sutures as compared with 63 percent of the controls.

---

[6]Constance Beynon, "The Normal Second Stage of Labour: A Plea for Reform in Its Conduct," *Journal of Obstetrics and Gynecology of the British Empire*, Vol. 64, No. 6, December 1957.

Constance Beynon first became interested in the spontaneous handling of second stage by noting that cardiac patients, who were not allowed to strain at all, delivered their babies just as easily and without any greater need for forceps than regular patients. She worked with her own patients in this way and then went on to do the study because people held on to the belief that a prolonged second stage or increased need for forceps would result from failure to push constantly.

It is difficult to believe, as Beynon states, "that about 80 percent of primigravid labours and most multiparous labours should come into the first category (completely normal). These patients are able to deliver themselves instinctively with little more straining than is required in the process of defaecation."[7] This is certainly different than our cultural norm!

So discuss this with your birth attendant, and make the choice to push only when you feel an *irresistible* urge and only as long as the urge remains during a contraction. Beynon concludes:

Not so long ago, obstetricians had to make a stand against the habit of an earlier generation of encouraging pushing from the very onset of labour. Everyone now accepts that pushing before full dilation is both useless and harmful and condemns it utterly. I make the plea that every stress above the minimum required in any given labour should now be regarded as unnecessary and unjustified risk to the tissues and therefore should also be vigorously condemned.[8]

WHEN YOU DO PUSH

The problem of when to push thus disappears. You push when the urge is irresistible and is taking you with it. Occasionally you will get a strong pushing urge when you are not yet fully dilated, and it is important to breathe through those contractions until dilation is complete. Don't resist the pushing urge in transition: allow it to be there, but continue to breathe through it just as you breathe through the tightening sensation of the contraction. It will feel as if your body is pushing, which is involuntary and is a sensation you should not run away from, but as long as you are breathing, you are not adding any extra force to these contractions before your cervix is completely opened (actively pushing against a partially dilated cervix can result in swelling, pain, and a longer labor).

By choosing not to push until you are fully dilated *and* have the powerful lead of your body, you rule out the possibility of a birth attendant misjudging dilation or friends (and you) wanting things to be further along than they are. Barring any abnormalities in position or

[7]*Ibid.*, p. 820.
[8]*Ibid.*

your pelvis, your baby will be born even if you give up on pushing (your uterus can push the baby out if you are relaxed and releasing your pelvic floor). If your attendant is anxious for more progress, squat during contractions, which will help bring the baby down and often increases the intensity of the pushing urge.

Of course, this approach to second stage does not mean that you can sit back and take a vacation. Second-stage contractions, although they may feel different from transition contractions, are usually quite strong, and your uterus is working very hard to push the baby out. If this is a first birth, you may have contractions that push the baby against your rectum for an hour or two as she descends. You will need to keep breathing to stay on top of the contractions and stay released, but you don't need to add active pushing effort (i.e., holding your breath and pushing with your diaphragm while bulging the pelvic floor) except when your body is involuntarily holding your breath for you. Don't breathe through the urge to push once you are fully dilated, but you needn't add anything extra except when your body is taking you with it.

POSITIONS FOR SECOND STAGE

So positions for second stage are the same as those for labor—propped up with lots of pillows, standing (leaning against your partner or the back of a chair), hands and knees, or squatting. About the only position you *won't* be using is the one routinely used in many hospitals—lying flat. When the head starts to be visible at the vaginal opening, you might want to lie back in a propped position with lots of pillows or with your coach behind you so your birth attendants can do perineal massage and aid with the gentle birth of the head. Let your legs flop apart, perhaps supported by pillows so you don't need to hold them at all. It's good for your perineal muscles if your feet are about fourteen inches apart. Let your arms relax at your sides. Keep your back and shoulders rounded and relaxed, jaw dropped slightly open. Feel the energy coming down through your head and out your vagina (untrained women tend to pull away from this energy and go backwards, out the back of their head). Consciously direct energy as you open. Your body and the energy of the Life Force are birthing your baby. Look over the bulge of your belly and see or touch the head as it begins to show. It's an exciting experience.

BULGING THE LOWER BELLY

When you are getting the urge to push with a strong second-stage contraction, there is something you can do to really help your body push effectively: bulge out your lower belly and perineum. Most of us, when we think of pushing as in having a bowel movement, think of pushing *in* on the belly as we hold our breath. This is just the opposite of what you need to do in second stage to birth your baby. Your baby's head requires that everything down below is open and stretches as the head bulges forward on your perineal tissues (see the photos of Mariposa's birth on pages 57–58).

Exercise 1 Have your husband place his hand on your lower belly and practice moving his hand out, as you did when practicing deep abdominal breathing.

Exercise 2 Now, with his or your hand pushed out by your belly, also push down with your pelvic floor muscles to bulge the entire lower belly and perineum (you should feel your vagina and anus wide open). Remember the "elevator" exercises from Chapter 2 in which you "went down into the basement?" This is the movement you want in pushing, so that everything is wide open for the baby to pass through. End by gently contracting the pelvic floor, so you leave the muscle with good tone.

Exercise 3 It's easier to do Exercises 1 and 2 while holding the breath, but this time, once you have bulged the lower belly and pelvic floor, hold them out and take several quick breaths to convince yourself that there is a definite independent muscular movement involved.

This bulging is important, for there is a tendency during strong second-stage contractions for the area just above the pubic bone to go in when the uterus hardens. You need to remember to counteract this tendency so your baby can come out more easily.

HOLDING THE BREATH

As the baby pushes against your lower bowel during descent, you will find that you start to get a catch in your breathing, and later on your breath will involuntarily be held. When your breath is held, your diaphragm (which goes across your body at the bottom of your ribs) is in a down position, pushing on the top of the uterus.

Feel what is happening with your body and don't strain unnecessarily. Holding your breath more than six or seven seconds has been shown to deprive your baby of oxygen. Many women don't hold the breath at all,

but push as they exhale, as they would in chopping wood or other exercise.

Exercise 1 Take a deep breath and hold it. Your diaphragm is pushing down on top of your uterus. This, together with bulging the pelvic floor, is all that is involved in pushing. Release the breath.

Exercise 2 Take a deep breath, hold it, and then drop your lower jaw. With your mouth open, you can still push. There's no need for chipmunk cheeks!

Exercise 3 Feel your stomach muscles while you blow into your fist like a trumpet. Even exhaling does not detract from the bearing-down effort.

RELAXING THE MOUTH

There is an unconscious neuromuscular association between the vagina and the mouth, so that if your pelvic floor muscles are tense (and they are often hard to relax when the baby is pushing against them), you can help to relax them by intentionally relaxing your mouth and jaw.

To demonstrate this connection, contract all the muscles of the pelvic floor, holding the vagina tightly closed. Feel your jaw, tongue and palate—you'll find that they have tension in them that can be released when you release the pelvic floor muscles. Similarly, clench your jaw, and tighten your lips and throat—now feel your vagina and see if it is relaxed and open. Almost everyone will have unconsciously contracted both.

This is why during labor, and especially during pushing, it is important to have the lower jaw dropped and the lips gently parted and loose. It is also why vomiting often increases dilation and the relaxation of the pelvic floor.

BREATHING THE BABY OUT

With a second baby the head may be visible at the vaginal opening before you ever push (so you don't need to push at all; your body will deliver the baby). But with a first baby you may have second-stage contractions for quite a while before the head is visible. This is normal, and it's important not to get discouraged. Also, the head will go back between contractions, but each time it will show a little more.

PRACTICING PUSHING CONTRACTIONS

Sit back against lots of pillows or sit supported by your partner (who then needs to be leaning against something comfortable). Let your legs flop apart. (Even though you may have been taught since the age of three to keep your legs together, you can't have a baby that way.) Your arms can be relaxed at your sides, your body rounded, jaw dropped, shoulders relaxed.

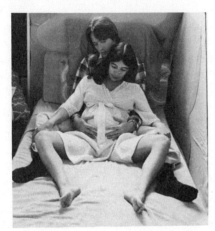

FIGURE 6-17. *Practice pushing with the legs well apart, shoulders and jaws relaxed.*

1. Contraction begins. Deep cleansing breath.
2. Feel the contraction build. Breathe as you normally do during contractions. When actually in a pushing contraction, you may find your breathing accelerates as the urge to push grows.
3. As the urge to push establishes itself strongly, inhale and hold the breath.

4. Then bulge the lower belly forward and the perineum out, opening the vagina. Coaches can help by putting a hand on your lower belly.
5. Check your shoulders and lower jaw—they should be rounded and relaxed.
6. When you run out of breath, feel the contraction again, perhaps taking several short breaths and then feeling the urge to hold again. In a really strong contraction, you may feel the urge to keep pushing through several held breaths. And then such a contraction might be followed by one or two weak ones.
7. When the contraction is over, take a deep cleansing breath and relax. After practicing contractions, contract your pelvic floor muscles gently so they always remain in good tone.

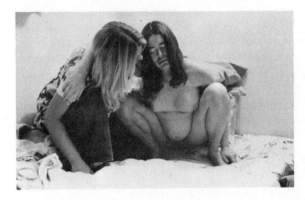

FIGURE 6-18. *Pushing while squatting.*

Try pushing in various positions. Think about opening up. Focusing on the opening rather than the contracting can help you remain relaxed both up top and down below, even when pushing.

As the head descends, it feels something like a grapefruit pressing down against the rectum and rounding the arch of your pubic bone. It's an amazing sensation, one you don't feel very many times! You may think, "How am I ever going to open up enough for the head to be born?" But with gradual stretching, the perineum does open to accommodate the head, which molds and makes itself as small as possible.

Once the baby's head can be seen, look over the curve of your belly, or have a large mirror so you can view the head as it comes further and further out. Reach down and touch it. Feel the amazing quality of the baby being both inside and outside at the same time. See and feel how strongly you need to push, and stop pushing when the perineum looks rigid and shiny or the head crowns (to minimize tearing).

As the baby starts to crown, you gradually feel your-self opening up, and you may get a warm, tingling sensation (like stretching the corners of your mouth very wide). Many prepared women find the crowning intensely pleasurable and very exciting. With a second or smaller baby, it is often possible to be sensitive to each part of the baby as it emerges from the birth canal.

By the time the head crowns (when the largest part stays at the vaginal opening), you should make sure you have stopped pushing and breathe through the contractions, no matter how strong the urge to push is. The force of your uterus alone is enough to bring your baby out. Adding extra force at this point can result in tearing of your tissue and isn't particularly good for the baby, either.

There is a tremendous feeling of release as the head slips out. Continue to breathe through the next contraction as the shoulders emerge, unless you are told by your

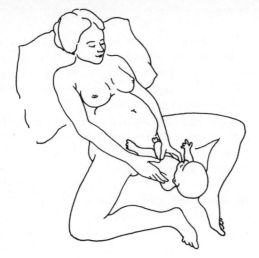

FIGURE 6-19.

attendant to give a gentle push. Again, if there has been no sign of fetal distress, it is not necessary to hurry this stage. Feel and savor it! Touch your baby, even before he is completely out, helping him to come up onto your belly once the shoulders are born (Figure 6-19).

FOCUSING DURING YOUR LAST SIX WEEKS OF PREGNANCY

Many things throughout your pregnancy contribute toward your preparation for the birth: regular exercise and good nutrition, practicing full-body relaxation when you have trouble sleeping, practicing breathing and relaxing when you're emotionally uptight, massaging your partner. Making sure that you're in good relationship with your partner affects how you feel and how you take care of yourself, as well as your experience of labor.

Because giving birth is not an exercise or an isolated event, I am reluctant to give a list of exercises. Your whole life is preparation. However, your last six weeks of pregnancy is a time to focus your energies, and to help with that, I am going to suggest some practices to aid you and your coach in communication and to put your attention on the upcoming birth.

Get into a comfortable position in bed, or on the floor, with lots of pillows. Make sure the room is warm enough and that no light is shining right in your eyes. Familiarize yourself with the exercises in this chapter.

EXPLORING RELAXATION

1. Coaches, talk her through whole body relaxation, starting at the eyes and working down through the whole body (p. 86).
2. Check and encourage her relaxation by lifting up her arms and legs in succession (p. 87).
3. Practice touch relaxation, so she releases to your hand (p. 87).
4. Reverse all of the above sometimes, and let her help *you* relax.

BREATHING WITH CONTRACTIONS

1. Call a contraction with your hand on her lower belly. Slow breathing should fill her body and move your hand (p. 90).
2. Do a contraction with light massage on her belly and upper thighs (p. 82).
3. Do a contraction in which she does light massage on herself. Remember, the breath should be slow and deep.
4. Do a contraction in the side relaxation position (p. 84).
5. Do a contraction while you push with steady pressure on her lower back, as in transition (p. 82).
6. Coach her through a really strong contraction using eye-to-eye contact (p. 83).
7. During one of the contractions, she might pull away or lose her breathing pattern. Have her blow out, establish eye contact, and breathe with her (p. 83).
8. Once or twice a week, simulate several contractions of varying strength by pinching the inside of her thigh; provide coaching to keep her relaxed (p. 87).
9. Help her into a squatting position and do a contraction.
10. Do a contraction standing up. Walk around. Do another.
• Always talk and hear her responses between contractions.

PUSHING WITH CONTRACTIONS

1. Help her into the contour position for pushing (p. 85).
2. Have her breathe with a contraction until she feels the urge to push just at the peak of it (p. 91). Remind her to (a) hold her breath, (b) bulge her lower belly, and (c) drop her shoulders and jaw. She resumes breathing once the pushing urge passes, until the contraction ends.
3. Repeat No. 2.
4. Now call a really strong contraction during which she will feel the urge to push for the entire contraction.
5. Repeat.
6. Now, during the contraction, tell her to stop pushing while the head crowns and is born (p. 91).

USING VISUALIZATIONS

Visualization can be a valuable tool in preparing for birth. Visualizations of normal labor and delivery can help your body and emotions to prepare in a way that bypasses the conscious brain. Done in a state of relaxation, they can increase your confidence in your body's knowledge and ability to give birth (just as it knows how to grow your baby). They can also be valuable tools for counteracting specific concerns from previous cesareans, for example. Many cassette tapes are available with guided visualizations, and several of the books listed on this page contain visualizations you may find helpful.

SELF-CHECK

1. Why is relaxation the key to labor?
2. What should you do if you can't get comfortable during labor?
3. Why do some women find clutching combs during contractions to be helpful?
4. What are the signs of hyperventilation? What should you do?
5. What can you do if you're feeling grumpy and complaining during labor?
6. What are the advantages and disadvantages of lying flat on your back, lying on your side, being in the contour position, standing, squatting?
7. Why is it important not to actively push before you're fully dilated?
8. When during a contraction should you push?
9. When pushing, what should you do with your
   - breath?
   - lower belly?
   - shoulders and jaw?
   - thoughts?
10. When should you *not* push?
11. Describe crowning:
    What is the baby doing?
    What is the mother doing?
    What is the coach doing?
    What is the birth attendant doing?

FOR FURTHER READING

Active Birth by Janet Balaskas. How to be in tune with your body and develop trust in your ability to birth.

Birthing Normally by Gayle Peterson. A valuable book with many visualizations and practical approaches to mind/body integration in childbirth preparation.

Childbirth Without Fear by Dr. Grantly Dick-Read. One of the classic works in the development of prepared natural childbirth. Emphasizes knowledge and relaxation to reduce pain.

The Experience of Childbirth by Sheila Kitzinger. Invaluable for her work with second stage, her exploration of relaxation and her discussion of psychosexual aspects of pregnancy and birth.

Husband-Coached Childbirth Dr. Robert Bradley. Addressed to the husband, this classic is valuable if you can handle his chauvinism.

Open Season by Nancy Cohen. *The* guide to natural childbirth and VBAC in the 90s.

Painless Childbirth by Dr. Fernand Lamaze. Lamaze's own explanation of the theory and practice of psychoprophylaxis.

Pregnancy as Healing by Gayle Peterson. More work with a holistic, mind/body approach to preparation for birth.

Pregnant Feelings by Rahima Baldwin and Terra Palmarini. Numerous exercises and visualizations for clearing the past and approaching birth with freedom and joy.

Silent Knife: Cesarean Prevention and Vaginal Birth after Cesarean by Nancy Cohen and Lois Estner. Detailed exploration of mindscapes and ways to prevent cesareans. Should be required reading.

Transformation Through Birth by Claudia Panuthos. Highly recommended for its exploration of the psychological aspects of pregnancy and birth. Excellent work with visualization.

CHAPTER SEVEN

Working Together During Labor and Delivery

This chapter is designed as a summary and easy reference for use during labor. It summarizes what the mother may be feeling and what she can do to help herself, what her coach can be doing to help, and what the birth attendant will be doing during the various stages of labor and delivery.

AS LABOR BEGINS

PHYSICAL SIGNS

• *Lightening*, felt as the baby drops when the head engages in your pelvis. Often a week or two before labor with first babies, not until labor with subsequent babies.

• Nesting urge and spurt of energy just before the birth. Don't redecorate the entire house!

• Weight loss, diarrhea, low-back pain, or an unusual feeling of pressure before labor begins. You may notice the baby is less active.

• You may be having contractions during your last month. If the contractions become stronger and closer together and don't stop when you walk, lie down, take a shower, etc., this may be labor beginning. Otherwise it's good practice.

• An increase in vaginal discharge is common, and you may notice the pinkish mucous plug come out. This *bloody show* is a sign that you will probably be in labor within 24 hours.

• The waters sometimes break with a gush or a trickle. Notify your birth attendant, and avoid vaginal exams or putting anything inside your vagina. Waters should be clear and odorless; you should be in active labor within 24 hours or be under close observation for infection.

FOR THE MOTHER

• Try to relax and nap each day during the last month. It's important to enter labor as well-rested as possible; it keeps your pain threshold high.

• Put time aside every day during your last month to work with your coach: feeling the baby, doing massage, working with breathing and relaxation.

• Gather your supplies together a month in advance; babies can easily arrive early.

• Make sure your emergency backup plan is complete and posted by the telephone.

• Babies can easily be late, too. Don't be thrown when you go past your due date—it's only a guide. Remain active to keep your mind from dwelling on it. Depression in the last month is actually more common than postpartum depression, so if you feel low try to give to your family or friends rather than dwelling on yourself. You won't be pregnant much longer!

• Notify your birth attendant if the waters break.

FOR HER PARTNER

The coach is usually the father, but a friend can also fill this role.

• Practice breathing and relaxation with her during the last month. She really needs to feel that you're involved and can be counted on.

• Make sure that your physical surroundings are as serene as possible. Try to avoid moving the last month!

• Make sure that the people who are coming to the birth know what they are going to do, are familiar with the process of birth, and understand what is important to the two of you (the kind of atmosphere you want, and so forth).

• Make sure your supplies are complete a month in advance and that your emergency backup is posted by the phone.

EARLY LABOR

If you are really in labor, your contractions will become stronger and closer together. Contractions may start a half hour apart, or they may begin five minutes apart (especially if the waters have ruptured). It's hard to predict, since each labor is different. Early labor (also called the latent phase) involves effacement (thinning out) and dilation (opening) of the cervix from 0 to 2½ centimeters. It is the longest phase, so don't be concerned with progress.

FOR THE MOTHER

• You'll probably find it very exciting actually to be in labor—it's the day you've been preparing for! Will you be able to handle it? Is everything together? What if you phone and your midwife doesn't answer? Calm down. Go through some whole-body relaxation; feel what is actually going on in your body and how strong the contractions are. Then, if it is the middle of the night, *go back to sleep!* You will need that extra energy at the end, especially if it is a long labor. Or, if it is during the day, continue with light activity.

• Walking and light activity tend to increase the effectiveness of labor. Lean on a countertop or against a wall or just put your attention on the breath as the contrac-

tions demand it. Otherwise, breathe normally as long as possible.

• As the contractions get stronger, place your attention on slow breathing, remembering the cleansing breaths at the beginning and end. Relax a little more with each outbreath.

• Decide whether you need an enema and do it now if you do. A full lower bowel will impede the baby's progress.

FOR HER PARTNER

• Help her with her relaxation, especially if she wakes you up or if you arrive home and find her in labor. Encourage her to release completely, using as slow a breathing rhythm as possible. Encourage her to rest or sleep if it is night, or to continue to be alert and focused outward if it is day and the contractions aren't too strong or too close. Hug and kiss a lot—it's a very special day.

• Time contractions occasionally, seeing how long they last and how far apart they are from beginning to beginning.

• Notify your birth attendants about the frequency of contractions, and alert friends who are going to be sharing with you. They may need to arrange child care, plan their day, etc.

• This is the longest stage. Unless contractions are three minutes apart and you can see the belly become hard during one, you probably aren't going to have a precipitous delivery!

• Check your supplies. Send someone to get anything you are missing: juices, food if your supplies are low, etc.

• Make sure that your environment is clean and serene to welcome the new being.

• If you have other children, make sure that someone will be present who can care for them and explain what is happening. You may get really busy later on!

• Make ice chips and frozen juice chips, and encourage her to eat small, light, easily digestible foods such as juices, blender drinks, soups, etc. It's important to keep her energy level up.

• Remind her to urinate every two hours.

FOR THE BIRTH ATTENDANT

• If you are there during early labor, note the strength of the contractions, and encourage her to stay relaxed and to breathe slowly.

• The "slumber party" atmosphere of early labor is best dispelled. Having her sleep or ignore labor helps it to progress. Leave the parents lots of opportunity for intimacy.

• Make certain that she urinates regularly.

• Palpate the position of the baby. Listen to the heart tones so you are familiar with their pattern. Check her blood pressure so you know what is normal for her. Review her prenatal records.

MIDDLE OR ACTIVE LABOR

The uterus is working harder now, opening to about 8 cms through contractions that are probably five minutes apart at first, decreasing to about three minutes apart or less. You may get a bloody show now. This is a good sign that labor is progressing. The waters may rupture.

FOR THE MOTHER

• You'll probably be feeling less outgoing now, having to concentrate more during each contraction.

• Relaxation is the key. Also important is communication with your coach, so he can help with massage, ice chips, etc.

• Use lots of pillows to form a contour position, or try walking or squatting if you feel up to it. Do some pelvic rocks if you have lower back pain. It may not be possible to get comfortable—you might have to just relax and breathe.

• Use the cleansing breath to release any tension that may have appeared during a contraction. Keep telling your body to release during contractions.

• Use positive statements of what you are trying to do. Give love to those around you and to the baby.

• Conserve your energy. Stay with slow, deep breathing which moves the stomach muscles, keeping them from becoming tense and painful when the uterus contracts.

• Stay focused in the present moment. Work with each contraction one at a time.

• Visualize your uterus opening up.

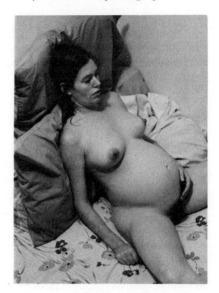

FIGURE 7-1. *Relaxing and concentrating during a contraction.*

FOR HER PARTNER

• Help her through encouragement and your loving touch.

• Help her to be more comfortable, remembering to get feedback as to what felt good and what she would like. Offer her pillows, blankets, ice or orange juice chips, a wet washcloth, sips of water, as needed. Try light massage on her belly and upper legs.

• Help her to stay in the present.

• Place your hand on her lower belly so she can feel it move with the breath. Keep her breathing slow and deep.

• Holding each other, kissing, and especially stimulating her breasts, all help to increase the energy of labor and can help her to feel really good, too.

• Maintain awareness of the entire room. If you want people to be more focused or less noisy, or to leave for a while, say so. Be aware of the energy level and the effect it and the individuals present may be having on the labor.

• Focus on the new being, welcoming the baby to the world without projecting about what he or she will be like.

- Feel what is happening with yourself. When was the last time you ate? Do you need a break or a short nap if there is someone else with whom she feels comfortable? She'll need you during transition!

FOR THE BIRTH ATTENDANT

- Spell the husband if he needs a break from coaching.

- Monitor the fetal heart tones every half hour.

- Keep a record of the labor (when heart tones are checked, etc.). See pages at the end of this section.

- Make sure the mother is staying relaxed and handling contractions well.

- Be aware of the quality of the interchange between the couple and the energy of other people present. Do what you feel will help the situation.

- **Remind her to urinate frequently; have her suck on orange juice chips or drink blender drinks to keep her energy level up.**

- Check the dilation if you think it will encourage her.

- If the waters break, make sure the fluid is clear, and check the fetal heart tones.

- Sterilize equipment for cutting the cord by boiling it for twenty minutes at a rolling boil; store in a covered casserole. Set up any other equipment.

TRANSITION

During transition the cervix is being pulled back over the baby's head, reaching 10 cm, or full dilation. The contractions are extremely intense. It is possible to see the belly harden during each contraction, and they may each have two or three peaks and be very close together. You may start getting some of the symptoms around 7 or 8 cms, or you may never notice you've been through it. Neither expect nor be surprised by it!

The waters will usually rupture if they haven't already, and there will be some bloody discharge (bloody show). The urge to push may start to be felt like the need to have a bowel movement or as a catching of the breath in the throat. It is important not to push until the cervix is completely opened.

FOR THE MOTHER

- You may experience one or two of the following symptoms which, together with the changing nature of

the contractions, can alert you that transition is approaching and that things are moving along very well. Some of these signs may occur several hours before full dilation, so don't get excited and lose your orientation of being in the present moment.

1. Nausea, vomiting, belching, hiccoughs
2. Hot and cold flashes, or feeling both at once
3. Trembling thighs
4. Restlessness, inability to get comfortable
5. Increased pressure or continuous backache
6. Not wanting to be touched (sensory overload)
7. Emotional rollercoastering; feeling discouraged, weepy, ecstatic, uncertain, or annoyed
8. Starting to feel the urge to push

- You can help yourself by staying focused on your coach during contractions.

- This is an especially good time to give energy to your coach and attendants and also to stay focused on the baby. Keep telling your body to release, paying special attention to the pelvic floor and legs, which tend to pull in and get trembly. Don't focus on your own discomfort or complain.

- Don't lie flat on your back! Try standing, supported by your coach or the back of a chair, or lie back with lots of pillows supporting you.

- Use the breathing technique that works for you. Staying with slow breathing takes real concentration, but it requires less energy and doesn't result in hyperventilation. If you are unable to keep your breathing slow and relaxed, it should be extremely light and shallow, using only your mouth. If you do feel dizzy or have tingling fingers, cup your hands over your nose and mouth and rebreathe your own air.

- Keep breathing through any urge to push in transition. Don't push until you are fully dilated with an irresistible urge to push.

FOR HER PARTNER

- Give her strong support: "I'm right here with you," "You're doing fine," etc. This is the time she needs you most, so don't leave her alone at this stage.

- Keep her in the present, working with each contraction individually. She may be getting discouraged and feel that labor will go on forever. Encourage her to rest between contractions.

- Use direct coaching and eye contact during contractions. Breathe with her, helping her to stay focused and keep in the rhythm.

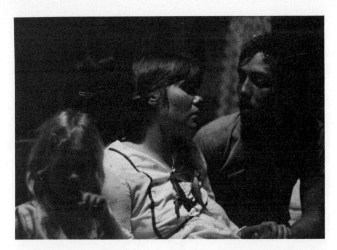

FIGURE 7-2. *Direct coaching during transition.*

• Watch carefully for wavering. If she loses her attention during a contraction, blow out with her and continue to breathe with her, maintaining eye contact.

• She probably won't feel like talking now; let a head or hand movement tell you what is comfortable. Things that felt good earlier may not feel good now.

• Wipe her face and neck with a cool washcloth. She will probably be perspiring and appreciate ice chips after a contraction.

• Use strong counterpressure on her sacrum (lower back) during contractions to counteract the pressure of the baby's head. Use your fist or the heel of your hand with steady, firm pressure.

• Massage the inside of her thighs if they start to tremble, or her calves if she gets leg cramps.

• Keep your confidence up. *You* may go through transition too. Remember that she really *can* do it, and once she is in second stage, her energy will come back.

• Keep her from pushing by keeping her breathing. If she is breathing she is not pushing, it's as simple as that. Encourage her to breathe through contractions until the pushing urge is overwhelmingly strong (she needs to avoid pushing before full dilation).

FOR THE BIRTH ATTENDANT

• Encourage the mother *and* the coach. Make sure she is staying on top of contractions through direct coaching. Help keep her focused.

• The fetal heart tones should be monitored every fifteen minutes in transition.

• Make sure that she urinates, as going into second stage with a full bladder can injure it and impede the baby's progress.

• Make certain when the waters break that they are clear and odorless. If they are stained with meconium, it is a sign of past or present fetal distress. Always check the heart tones when the waters break. The bloody show will occur, similar to menstrual bleeding.

• Check dilation once the pushing urge establishes itself. Even after dilation is complete, she should have a strong pushing urge before she pushes.

SECOND STAGE: DESCENT AND BIRTH

The strong contractions which have completely opened the uterus now push your baby down the birth canal and out the vaginal opening into the world. The contractions feel quite different than they did in transition. There is a longer rest between them and your energy usually comes back. It is an exciting stage, and not as uncomfortable as transition may have been.

FOR THE MOTHER

• Once you are fully dilated, continue to breathe through contractions, pushing only as long and as hard as each contraction dictates. You may feel only a small stopping of your breath, or you may feel the irresistible urge to push for the entire contraction. Let your body guide you.

• Assume whatever position feels good to you (except lying flat, which necessitates your baby's moving "uphill"). Squatting during contractions opens the pelvis and the birth canal. Or sit propped up with pillows, or with your partner behind you.

• Once the head is visible at the vaginal opening, you might want to sit with your legs flopped apart so your attendants can do perineal massage to prevent tearing.

• Once you are fully dilated, work with the urge to push. Hold your breath or exhale with it, bulging your lower belly and perineum. Remember to keep your shoulders relaxed and your jaw open.

• Feel yourself opening like a giant flower. Don't resist the sensations. Give in to the energy which is flowing through you and birthing your baby. There's no need to strain. During a contraction, think about the energy flowing in the direction the baby is moving.

• Stay focused on the baby, the real purpose of pushing. Give him love. Watch the head as it appears at the vaginal opening. Touch it if you want to.

• When the head starts to crown you'll feel a stretching and possibly a burning sensation. STOP PUSHING by doing light breathing.

• Breathe the baby out slowly. Relate with the baby as he comes out. Watch in the mirror, or reach down and touch him. There's no reason why you can't touch him or help to bring him up on your belly if he doesn't have difficulty breathing.

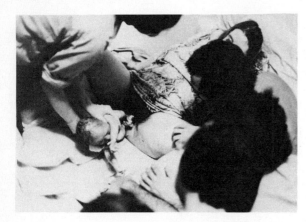

FIGURE 7-3.

FOR HER PARTNER

• Encourage her that the contractions will bring the baby down and that she has plenty of room.

• Remind her to relax her pelvic floor (check her jaw and throat to see that they are relaxed).

• Encourage her to breathe through contractions until the pushing urge is holding her breath involuntarily. While that happens, encourage her lower belly to bulge forward, check that her shoulders and jaw are rounded and relaxed, and encourage her to open.

• Encourage her to keep her eyes open and participate in what she's doing. Remind her to direct energy down through her head and out the vagina.

• Help her to relax fully between contractions. There is usually a longer rest period between contractions than there was in transition. Take advantage of it!

• Once the head crowns, get her to stop pushing by doing light breathing with her. Help to keep things calm and let her calmly breathe the baby out. Convey the instructions of the attendant to her.

• As the baby is born, think of his experience. You may want to have someone dim the lights and make sure everyone is calm and quiet as the head comes out. Encourage your birth attendant to put the baby immediately onto the mother's belly if he isn't having difficulties.

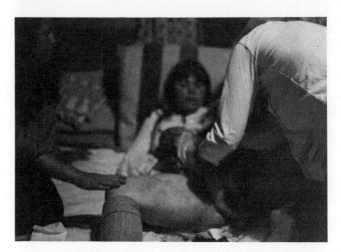

FIGURE 7-4. *Putting the baby on the mother's belly immediately.*

FOR THE BIRTH ATTENDANT

• Monitor the fetal heart tones (midwifery texts recommend every ten minutes).

• Don't encourage her to push any more than her body is telling her to push. If you become concerned about lack of progress after an hour, you might try having her squat.

• When she is pushing, encourage her to release the pelvic floor.

• Once the head is stretching the perineum, massage the vaginal opening with fresh olive oil or apply hot sterile compresses to the perineum. The aim is to let the birth of the head be gradual and prevent tearing.

• Have the lights dimmed and radiate calm as the head starts to crown. Instruct the mother to breathe through these final contractions.

• Once the head is out, check to see if the cord is wrapped around the baby's neck. If so, you can probably hook a finger under it and loop it over the baby's head. If not, try to loosen it and loop it over the shoulders as they come out. If the cord is extremely tight or too short, or the baby goes into distress and doesn't come out any further with the next contractions, tie the cord in two places and cut immediately. Have the mother push, even between contractions, and be prepared to resuscitate the baby if necessary.

• If there was meconium in the water, or if the baby was born persistent posterior (face up), the mouth and nose should be suctioned as soon as the head is out. With meconium staining the back of the throat and trachea should be suctioned with a DeLee suction catheter and the baby watched for respiratory problems. Otherwise, you can wait and see if the baby is particularly mucousy before suctioning with a bulb syringe.

• The head is usually born face down and will rotate back to the side by itself. Just support it. Note which side it turns toward.

• There may be a couple of minutes until the next contraction. Then gently support the baby and the perineum as the top shoulder is born.

• The bottom shoulder will be born right after the top and the body will follow without any difficulty.

• Someone should note the time of the birth (when the whole body is out).

• Put the baby up onto the mother's stomach.

• Pay close attention to the baby. If it is especially mucousy and has trouble breathing, suction mouth and nose with a bulb syringe.

• Listen for the baby's breath, allowing it to come naturally. Remember to breathe yourself. The baby should start to breathe and pink up within a minute or so. Otherwise you can stimulate the baby through touch and begin resuscitation if it seems necessary. If the baby is white and limp, do cardiopulmonary resuscitation immediately (Chapter 8).

• Be attentive to the baby, doing an Apgar Score at one minute and at five minutes (i.e., note if anything is not excellent).

• Allow the mother and father to massage and caress the baby while it is on her belly. Cover it with a receiving blanket if the room is not very warm.

• Once the cord has stopped pulsing and is white and limp (usually about 5 to 10 minutes), it can be tied about one to two inches from the baby's umbilicus and again an inch beyond that, and cut between the two ties. Let the parents cut the cord. Use sterile clamps or ties and scissors.

• If the parents wish to follow LeBoyer's example of placing the baby in a warm-water bath, someone should bring a clean baby bathtub with water that is deep enough to cover the baby's body so he won't become chilled. The water should be body temperature (about 99°F). It should be placed where the mother can see and participate while the father gently holds the baby in the water.

THIRD STAGE: THE PLACENTA

Once the baby is in your arms, you'll feel much less tired than you did earlier and will be amazed at the entire miracle of birth. Reassure and welcome your baby with your loving touch and enjoy being with him or her. Nursing right away stimulates the production of oxytocin, which causes uterine contractions, thus aiding the expulsion of the placenta and preventing hemorrhage.

FOR THE MOTHER

• When you feel the next contractions or when the cord lengthens, squat over a bowl to deliver the placenta. Usually the placenta comes within twenty minutes after the birth.

• Let the baby nurse frequently to keep your uterus contracted. Be in a comfortable position and stroke the baby's cheek with your finger or nipple. He will turn toward the sensation and start to "root" for the nipple, searching with an open mouth. Place the nipple and the areola in the baby's mouth so he can latch on and start nursing. You may need to hold your finger between the baby's nose and your breast to make an air passage. Stay comfortable and relaxed.

• Drink lots of fluids to counteract body loss. Have a good meal if you're hungry. Don't get up too soon, and have help. Get some sleep. Congratulations!

FOR HER PARTNER

• Enjoy yourselves as a new family! Do the LeBoyer bath together if it seems that the baby would like it. Savor each moment.

• Praise her handling of the birth and help her squat over a bowl for the expulsion of the placenta (or be with the baby while your attendant does this and helps her to get cleaned up and comfortable again).

FOR THE BIRTH ATTENDANT

• Once the baby has started to breathe, turn your attention back to the mother.

• Watch for the lengthening of the cord and a gush of blood, signals that the placenta has come away. Get the mother up into a squatting position to deliver the placenta (or have her squat if she feels any contractions).

• See that the uterus feels firm and watch for excessive bleeding or signs of shock, especially if the placenta does not come out within the first half hour. Use nipple stimulation, a squatting position, or have her sit on the toilet and relax to try to get it to come out.

• Massage the uterus every fifteen minutes during the first hour after the placenta is out to make sure it is hard and below the umbilicus.

• Keep watching the mother for excessive bleeding.

• Examine the placenta and membranes to make sure they are complete. Get a sample of cord blood if the mother is Rh negative.

• Estimate the amount of blood, once it separates from the amniotic fluid in the bowl. Add in the amount on the sheets and pads; the total should be less than two cups.

• Get her to drink juice or eat.

• Let the family have time together to experience themselves as a new family.

• Examine the mother's vulva and perineum, using sterile gloves and a good light, to see if she has torn and will require suturing.

• See that the mother gets cleaned up. She should always have someone with her in the bathroom.

• See that the baby's needs are met. Check the baby to make sure there are no difficulties or abnormalities. The baby doesn't need to be scrubbed—the vernix is really good for the skin and can be rubbed in. You might weigh the baby with the parents participating, and ask them if they are going to use drops in the eyes.

• Advise them on postpartum care and answer their questions. Tell them where they can contact you during the next few hours. Visit the new family several times in the next few days. Encourage the mother to have people come in and help with the cleaning, laundry, shopping, and so forth.

POINTS TO REMEMBER DURING LABOR

FIRST STAGE

• There is no blueprint for labor. Accept your own pattern. Be informed and prepared, but don't be trapped by your expectations of how it will be. Stay in the here-and-now and deal with each contraction one at a time.

• Feel! Say "yes" to sensation. Feel what is going on with your body. Trust your body and its ability to give birth. Allow the Life Force to flow through you. You can control yourself, but not your labor. Welcome its increasing intensity and the birth of your baby.

• Remember to sleep if possible during early labor. Despite your excitement, you'll really need the energy later. Light activity, walking, sitting, or squatting help labor to progress, but lie down if you feel tense.

• Relaxation is the key to labor. Do whole-body relaxation. Use the breath to relax more deeply.

• During contractions, tell your body to release, and stay centered in slow, deep breathing. Keep your eyes open and stay focused on what you are doing.

• Pay attention to the baby, creating a loving environment into which he can be born. Saying "I love you" to the baby or to your husband can help open you up. Give to the people around you, being thankful and courageous.

• Use positive statements with yourself. Say what you are trying to do (e.g., "I'm opening up" or "I'm relaxing more and more"). Don't complain, but voice any questions, fears or thoughts you may have and get them cleared up.

SECOND STAGE

• Feel and breathe with each contraction and push only as hard and as long as it dictates.

• Keep your chin down, shoulders and jaw relaxed.

• Cooperate with any sensations of bulging or stretching.

• Think about opening, and feel the energy coming down through your head and out your vagina with each contraction.

• When you are told to stop pushing, do light breathing as your baby is born.

Remember, there is no standard to be achieved. There is no such thing as failure in labor. Go with your own pattern of labor, contraction by contraction. Each one is moving you nearer the birth of your baby.

RECORD OF LABOR AND DELIVERY

Position of the baby at last prenatal exam (date): _____

Position of baby at beginning of labor (by palpation): _____

Fetal heart tones: _____ Mother's blood pressure: _____

When did the waters break (date, time)? _____

    Any color or odor? _____

    Fetal heart tones checked then? (rate) _____

Timing Contractions: It isn't necessary to record *every* contraction. Do it from time to time to see how things are progressing. Note the time at the beginning and end of a contraction. Subtract the two to figure the duration (how long it lasted) and subtract the starting time of this one from the starting time of the next one to calculate the frequency ("how often" is figured from beginning to beginning).

Things to watch for: Keep a record of the fetal heart tones, when the mother urinates, symptoms of transition, the beginning of second stage, the effectiveness of contractions, dilation and station of the head if they are checked vaginally. Always note the time as well.

Date/ Time	Frequency of Contraction	Length of each Contraction	FHT	Dilation	Blood Pressure	NOTES

Date/ Time	Frequency of Contraction	Length of each Contraction	FHT	Dilation	Blood Pressure	NOTES

BIRTH RECORD

Parents' names: _____

Address: _____

Baby's name: _____ Sex: _____

Date: _____ Time: _____ Weight: _____

Birth attendant(s): _____

Others present: _____

_____

Apgar Score: At 1 minute   At 5 minutes
   Color
   Muscle tone
   Breathing
   Heart rate
   Reflex response
    Total

When did the baby breathe? _____
  Did it require any assistance (what)? _____

Length of Labor: 1st Stage _____ 2nd Stage _____
               3rd Stage _____ _____

Mother's condition after the birth, and her reactions: _____
_____

How long until the cord was cut? _____ Who cut it? _____

Signs of placental separation (include approximate time):
  Lengthening of the cord: _____
  Cord stops pulsating: _____
  Gush of blood: _____
  Rise and mobility of the uterus: _____

Delivery of the placenta (time): _____
  Mother's position: _____
  Anything done to help it happen: _____
  Placenta complete (both sides): _____
  Membranes complete: _____
  Any cord abnormalities: _____

Amount of blood lost: _____
  If an abnormal amount, describe bleeding: _____
  Measures taken: _____

Using sterile technique, check for tears: _____

Other notes: _____
_____
_____

NOTES

THE BIRTH OF FAITH RAINBOW

Rahima

Before I became pregnant with Faith I was determined to solve the questions I had about "painless" childbirth, so I trained as a childbirth educator with the Childbirth Education Association of Los Angeles (modified Lamaze technique). Just as I finished the course we moved to Cuernavaca, Mexico, where Wahhab and I had been asked to open a Sufi Center.

Once we had learned Spanish and the center was under way, I began teaching Lamaze classes in Spanish in order to share the good news of prepared childbirth and to learn more about birth in Mexico. It was quite a different experience to teach in a culture where there was no recognition that prepared birth was possible. Birth was expected to be painful, and anyone with education or money wanted to deliver in the hospital with anesthetics so they wouldn't have to suffer so much.

We became close friends with Margaret and Jenny and their friends and I heard their account of Mariposa's birth without the aid of a doctor. I was amazed, appalled, aghast, fascinated; I had numerous arguments and discussions with them during the months that followed. But by the time we were ready to have our second baby, both of us were ready to take responsibility for the birth in many ways that we hadn't done with Seth's.

We undertook Faith's conception and birth, like Seth's, as an act of service in response to a spiritual prompting. This time I became pregnant the first month. Faith, like Seth, was born ten days early, on Seth's original due date, two years later.

By the time my due date was approaching, our ideas had changed sufficiently that we knew we wanted Wahhab to catch the baby. I had been seeing Susannah, a midwife of Japanese/Mexican heritage, during the pregnancy. She had never seen a prepared birth, but had read about them, and when I gave her the Spanish version of *Birth Without Violence* she was so excited that she tried it with her very next delivery. I liked her a lot and wanted to share the birth with her. And even though I knew that the birth would go completely smoothly, I still felt good having her there in case anything should happen.

About ten days before my due date, I awoke at 6 A.M. with the breaking of the waters. After the initial excitement, and realizing that this time I wasn't having any contractions, I gathered together everyone at the center after breakfast and gave them a crash course in normal labor and delivery and what we were going to be doing. I felt that this wasn't *my* baby, but a birth to share with all my friends. Contractions still didn't materialize, so everyone went about their daily schedule. I walked around a lot, dripping water, but still with no contractions.

By the time I went to sleep around 10 P.M. contractions were fifteen minutes apart. I slept until contractions woke me at one, occurring strongly every five minutes. We assembled everyone and Susannah came at two to check dilation. I was only 2 cm, so she said she would come back in the morning. I'd been through that movie before!

But this time I didn't feel at all discouraged and things took a new twist—my body started to shake. I had so much energy flowing through me that six people stayed around me just to lay their hands on me and try to absorb it all. Contractions were welcome, because they stopped the shaking! A friend was at my head, breathing with me, and everyone else was so supportive. Wahhab was free to walk around, beaming from ear to ear, looking beatific. I felt so loved and cared for, and was immensely grateful to have so many people to share with me and help me.

Within two hours I could feel Faith moving down, and I told Wahhab that if Susannah was going to make this birth she had better appear soon. I knew exactly what my body was doing, and I never pushed as I felt Faith coming down the birth canal. My eyes were wide with amazement and I could feel myself opening—it's such a powerful sensation. I was grinning; it was incredible. Wahhab was catching Faith just as Susannah walked in the door. He whispered in the baby's ear, "*La ilaha ill'Allah* (There is no god but God), but in the meantime your name is Faith Rainbow Baldwin" and put her immediately up on my belly.

The birth had been completely without tightening or shock for either Faith or me. She was totally aware, without any tension or constriction. When we contemplated putting her in warm water, it was clear that she didn't need it and that it would interrupt what she was already experiencing. So I just kept holding her.

Wahhab cut the cord, and the placenta came without any problems. Susannah couldn't stop raving about the birth. She had never seen a baby come out so smoothly; it was clear to her that something special was going on.

I hadn't torn, had only a few days of bleeding afterwards, and felt fantastic. I was up and about the next day and had to keep telling myself not to overdo it. It was wonderful living in a community of so many caring people. And it was really good for Seth, too, because he never experienced jealousy of Faith. Since there were so many adults around, his world didn't change as much as it would have in a nuclear family. The birth had been at 4:30 A.M., so he had been asleep, but in the morning he circled around me without saying good morning for about a minute and then formed an immediate and deep relationship with his sister. We always let him love and hold her, with support, and we were really pleased by the immediate bonding that occurred between the two of them.

The birth was a very high experience, and I felt completely fulfilled. We had taken responsibility for the birth and wouldn't have done anything differently. We were really grateful that Faith could be born so easily and with so much joy.

CHAPTER EIGHT

Complications and Emergencies

This chart is designed as both a table of contents for this chapter and as a quick reference to the signs of complications which may occur during the various stages of labor. The complications discussed in this chapter are those not likely to be predicted in advance; for complications of pregnancy which are predictable in advance, see Chapter 2.

COMPLICATIONS AND EMERGENCIES

The great majority of all labors and births go along completely normally. Moreover, with good prenatal care, 85 percent of all complications can be predicted in advance. However, some labors will develop problems, and it is especially important in a homebirth situation that these be recognized and acted upon. This chapter gives an outline of things that can arise in homebirth, along with a summary of emergency measures that your birth attendant can take, as well as some discussion of your options in the hospital.

What is the chance that you will have a problem of some kind? Of course your own body, your prenatal care, diet and exercise will uniquely determine this for you. But in Holland, which has an excellent system of home delivery, it is estimated that 8 percent of first-time homebirth mothers and 2 percent of repeat mothers go to the hospital during labor, delivery or postpartum.[1] And in a study of 1046 women in California beginning labor at home with the intention of delivering there, 136 (11.9 percent) were sent to the hospital for treatment of intrapartum (11 percent) or postpartum (0.9 percent) problems.[2] Fortunately, very few homebirths that do involve a trip to the hospital have time-pinch emergencies. They are most often for some complication about which your birth attendant does not feel confident or that requires more equipment and procedures than are available at home.

WHEN DO YOU GO TO THE HOSPITAL?

Many of the variations in labor, although they might be termed complications since they are variations from the norm, will not require medical treatment if maternal and fetal signs remain good. Other complications may require a trip to the hospital, but with plenty of time. Some complications, such as tearing, could be handled at home depending on the skills of your birth attendant. But there are a few genuine emergencies which require immediate action and getting to the hospital as quickly as possible.

It is important to know what these are, to recognize their symptoms and to be able to act on them quickly. Of course, this is one of the values of having a skilled birth attendant. A birth attendant's experience of handling many births will help her to know which situations are abnormal; the fact that the parents are so intimately involved in this birth and have seen so few others may make it very difficult for them to examine a possible complication with sufficient dispassion to maintain clarity and a correct diagnosis.

At the same time, the intuition of the parents, especially the mother, must not be ignored. If the mother feels she should go to the hospital and direct coaching doesn't dispel this feeling, TAKE HER TO THE HOSPITAL. She may not be in any condition to give a rational discourse on why she should or shouldn't go, but she knows her own body. Trust that knowledge.

Sometimes it is very clear that you need to go to the hospital, and other times it is a difficult decision to make. Discuss the situation with your attendant and each other so you feel that you are making the best decision for the safety and well-being of mother and baby.

COMPLICATIONS OF THE ONSET OF LABOR

PROLONGED RUPTURE OF THE MEMBRANES

1. Symptom: Waters have broken, but 24 hours later the baby has not yet delivered.

2. Incidence: Water ruptures first in about 10 percent of births. At term, 95 percent do go into labor within 24 hours.

3. Danger of infection, but incidence isn't higher if there are no vaginal exams. Baby can become infected without signs.

4. What to do:
   a. If waters are brown or green or foul-smelling, see your attendant immediately (baby may be in distress, have infections, etc.).
   b. If waters are clear, notify your attendant and confidently relax.
   c. Don't put anything inside the vagina—you are both vulnerable to infection.
   d. If you don't go into labor, your doctor may want to induce, or may let it go another day while monitoring your temperature and white blood cell count and/or giving you antibiotics.
   e. If waters leak several weeks early, it is possible they can reseal. Notify your attendant to monitor for infection; bed rest recommended.
   f. If you're birthing in hospital, stay home until labor is established.

PREMATURE LABOR

1. Definition for homebirth: Labor starting 2½ weeks or more before a known due date.

---

[1]G. J. Kloosterman, "Obstetrics in the Netherlands: a Survival or a Challenge?" delivered at the Meiu Tunbridge Wells Meeting, 1975.

[2]Lewis Mehl et al., "Outcomes of Elective Home Birth: A Series of 1046 Cases" presented before the North American Society of Psychosomatic Obstetrics and Gynecology, April 10, 1976, Chicago, Illinois.

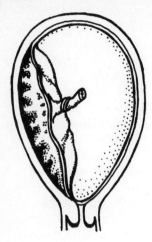 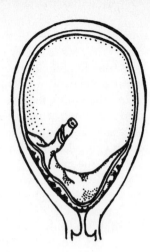

Figure 8-1. *(a) Low-lying placenta, and (b) placenta covering the opening of the cervix.*

2. Incidence: 10 percent of American labors are after 36 weeks or less of pregnancy.

3. Danger: Babies have more trauma in labor, are less developed and usually require intensive care.

4. What to do:
    a. If you don't think it's early, have your due date, size of baby, and when you conceived re-evaluated by your attendant.
    b. If you are 1 cm or less dilated and there has been no bloody show and the waters are intact, a glass of wine may stop contractions. Go to bed in a quiet environment; when there are no contractions for 24 hours, get up for a little as long as no contractions ensue. In the hospital, terbutaline or ritoerine would be prescribed.
    c. If your baby is several weeks early the risks may advise against birthing at home.
    d. If your baby is born prematurely in the hospital, see page 126.

Going Past Your Due Date

1. Incidence: Only 5 percent of women deliver on their due date; it is not uncommon to be one or even two weeks early or late.

2. Danger: Stillbirth rate is high; larger, more calcified head can result in more difficult labor and increased trauma to baby; placental insufficiency can endanger the baby. Meconium aspiration and hypoglycemia are more common.

3. If more than 2½ or 3 weeks late, consider placental sufficiency and the risks of homebirth. If you don't go into labor, induction with pitocin is usual, or a cesarean if that doesn't work.

_____
[3]Dr. and Mrs. Fritz Fuchs' studies of this were quoted in "Medicine," *Time*, February 9, 1968.

4. What to do:
    a. Consider your due date: when did you conceive, menstrual and gestational history, size of baby.
    b. Have placental sufficiency tests to evaluate estriol level; nonstress test records heart tones and movement.
    c. If there are still questions, biophysical profiles may be done with ultrasound.
    d. Having your spine adjusted or acupuncture can bring on labor. Or take one tablespoon of castor oil in the morning (you'll either get labor or the runs.) Try nipple stimulation.
    e. Don't let anyone use pitocin or rupture your membranes to induce labor at home. Don't do a pitocin stress test in the hospital unless you're ready to have an induced labor or a cesarean.

COMPLICATIONS OF FIRST STAGE (LABOR)

Bright Red Bleeding During Labor

1. Definition: The bloody show during active labor is normal and is a sign of progress. It is a dark, mucousy discharge. But a mother bleeding fresh, bright red blood during first stage labor is an emergency.

2. DANGER! EMERGENCY! CALL AMBULANCE OR RUSH TO HOSPITAL. If she is in shock, keep her on her back with legs elevated. Have someone phone ahead to the hospital so they can prepare for a cesarean. Give oxygen.

3. Possible placenta praevia (low-lying placenta).
    a. May be just low-lying (Figure 8-1a) or partially or completely covering the opening of the cervix (Figure 8-1b); uterus is not painful.
    b. Incidence: 1 in 200-400 births; associated with age, multiparity, malpresentation and other risk factors.
    c. Do not do vaginal exam—may induce massive hemorrhage.
    d. Cesarean section most likely.
    e. If bleeding in late pregnancy, may be diagnosed by sonogram.

4. Possible abruptio placentae (premature separation of the placenta).
    a. May be with vaginal bleeding (80 percent of cases) (Figure 8-2a) or may be concealed hemorrhage behind the placenta (20 percent of cases) (Figure 8-2b).
       (1) Uterus may be painful and tender and/or boardlike and hard, or enlarged with blood.

(2) Drop in blood pressure of ten points or more (diastolic pressure) may be the first sign.

(3) Fetal heartbeat may be slowed or absent.

(4) Mother may show signs of shock (see next item).

b. Incidence: 1 in 420 pregnancies, but less common in low-risk mothers. Often manifests in second or third trimester; more likely with grand multiparity, twins, toxemia, chronic hypertension.

c. Immediate c-section necessary to save mother and baby; no vaginal exam except in operating room. If separation is over a large area, the baby may die, whether in a home or hospital birth. This is probably the worst emergency that can occur. If there is only partial separation, the baby should receive enough oxygen to get to the hospital. No eating or drinking prior to general anesthesia.

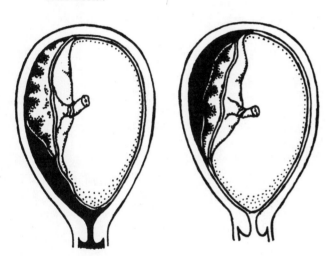

FIGURE 8-2. *(a) Abruptio placenta with vaginal bleeding, and (b) with hidden hemorrhage.*

SHOCK

1. Know the symptoms of shock:
   a. Pale skin, cold sweat.
   b. Low body temperature; chills; shaking in bad cases.
   c. Feeble pulse, over 90/minute.
   d. Drop in blood pressure more than ten points or low blood pressure (systolic less than 100, unless her normal has been less than that).
   e. May include restlessness, anxiety or unconsciousness.

2. Caused by bleeding; can be compounded by anemia, dehydration or fear.

3. EMERGENCY! CALL AMBULANCE OR RUSH TO HOSPITAL WITH MOTHER ON BACK, LEGS ELEVATED. Keep her warm (but not flushed). Give her liquids if she is conscious and able to drink (1 tsp. salt and ½ tsp. baking soda dissolved in 1 qt. water). Give oxygen.

MOTHER NOT COPING BETWEEN CONTRACTIONS: MATERNAL DISTRESS

1. Possible causes and what to do:
   a. Check for signs of shock (above): RUSH TO HOSPITAL.
   b. Possible dehydration and electrolyte imbalance. Prevent by eating and drinking—expecially runner's drink. Should go to hospital: IF THE MOTHER ISN'T DOING WELL, THE BABY CAN'T DO WELL EITHER. Usual treatment is IV drip, and/or pain medication.
   c. Fever, foul-smelling amniotic fluid: TO HOSPITAL. Infection, damage to baby.
   d. Physical exhaustion from a prolonged labor, or beginning labor in a weakened condition (after flu, etc.); can give oxygen if birth is imminent and baby is fine; otherwise to hospital due to danger of maternal and fetal distress and postpartum hemorrhage from an exhausted uterus.
   e. Mother not handling contractions, wants to go to hospital. If transition, remind her that everything is all right and she'll be in second stage soon. If direct coaching does not bring her through the problem and she still wants to go to the hospital, she should. Extreme pain or pain when pushing can be an indication of some other problem and should be checked out.

AMNIOTIC FLUID BROWN OR GREEN

1. Indicates the baby has passed meconium from his intestines due to lack of oxygen causing relaxation of the anal sphincter. Dangerous if postmature.

2. Incidence: 5 to 10 percent of all births. Mortality rate is less than 1 percent with clear fluid; 6 percent perinatal mortality with meconium staining.

3. Go to hospital if:
   a. Heartbeat is irregular, around 110 or above 160.
   b. Meconium is "pea-soup green"; thick or clumpy.
   c. Waters are foul-smelling (probably infection).

4. If the heartbeat is strong and regular, and meconium is light, it is a sign of past momentary distress. If the heartbeat remains good, a good delivery is possible. The danger is that the baby might inhale the meconium and develop meconium inhalation pneumonitis, which can prevent him from getting enough oxygen and result in death. If

you decide to continue the birth at home, suction baby's nose and mouth thoroughly as soon as head is out to prevent meconium going into lungs. If your attendant has a DeLee suction trap it should be used. Watch for respiratory distress; if present see pediatrician or hospital without delay.

BABY'S HEARTBEAT LOW OR RACING: FETAL DISTRESS

1. Sign: fetal heart tones (FHT) around 110 (very serious if 100 or below) or around 180 between contractions, or count varying widely, or weak and irregular.
   a. FHT should be monitored every half hour during labor, every 15 minutes during transition and every 10 minutes during pushing.
   b. Always listen for the FHT when the waters break to make sure the cord has not prolapsed.
   c. If heartbeat is around 110 or above 160, listen during and immediately after a contraction. Heartbeat will slow during contraction but should pick up right away. If it is slow after contraction, further sign of distress!
2. DANGER TO THE BABY: fetal distress means baby isn't getting enough oxygen. Can lead to brain damage and death.
3. What to do. Give the mother oxygen and:
   a. If the birth is imminent, keep pushing while lying on left side or squatting to get the baby out as quickly as possible (perhaps with episiotomy); cardiopulmonary resuscitation (CPR) if necessary.
   b. If distress occurs when the waters break, put mother in the knee-chest position and GO TO THE HOSPITAL (see prolapsed cord under next heading).
   c. If distress occurs in first stage of labor, get onto your left side (best position for circulation to the baby) and recheck heartbeat.
   d. If the left side doesn't help, get into knee-chest position (see Figure 8-3.). Recheck heartbeat. Check vaginally for prolapsed cord (see next heading). If heartbeat doesn't become regular and strong, or if you feel the cord, GO TO THE HOSPITAL! In the hospital, they will monitor the situation and see if a cesarean is necessary for the safety of the baby.
4. Some possible causes:
   a. Condition of the baby (pre- or post-mature; knotted cord very rare).
   b. Precipitous delivery (total labor two hours or less).

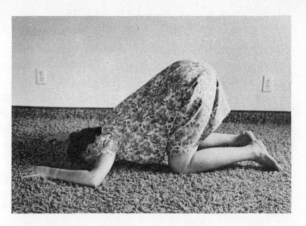

FIGURE 8-3. *Knee-chest position for emergencies.*

   c. Prolonged labor, especially with lack of progress.
   d. Anemia in the mother, high blood pressure, toxemia, or anesthesia.
   e. Premature rupture of the membranes with infection.
   f. Abruptio placentae (placenta coming away from uterus).
   g. Prolapsed cord.

CORD IN OR OUTSIDE OF VAGINA: PROLAPSED CORD

1. The cord is prolapsed when it comes down before the baby once the waters have broken (Figures 8-4a and 8-4b) or if it is pinched between the head and the pelvis (Figure 8-4c).
2. Incidence: 1 in 1,500 if your baby is head down. Incidence much greater with breech or transverse lie, hydramnios or multiparity (especially when the head is not engaged).

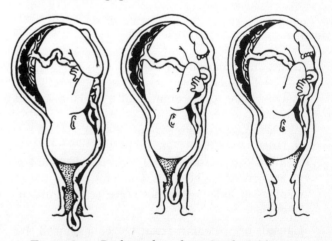

FIGURE 8-4. *Prolapsed cord. (a) Cord visible outside the vagina, (b) cord in vagina, and (c) hidden prolapse.*

3. DANGER TO THE BABY of intrauterine death through compressing blood and oxygen supply.

4. If you see or feel the cord or suspect a hidden prolapse through slowing of the fetal heart tones, put the mother in KNEE-CHEST POSITION (see accompanying photo).
   a. Using a long sterile glove, put your hand in the vagina and see if you feel the cord and/or can lift up the head off the cord, especially during contractions.
   b. If you feel the cord, or if this technique brings back the heartbeat, transport the mother TO THE HOSPITAL—with your hand inside if you are restoring the heartbeat.
   c. If the cord is outside the vagina, do not handle it. Wrap it loosely in a warm, moist gauze or cloth to keep it warm and prevent spasm.
   d. Give the mother oxygen.
   e. Phone ahead with details so the hospital can prepare for a cesarean section.

ENTIRE LABOR LIKE TRANSITION: PRECIPITOUS DELIVERY

1. Labors lasting two hours or less often have extremely intense contractions.

2. What to do:
   a. Watch for increased risk of fetal distress.
   b. Give direct coaching.
   c. Set up your equipment NOW.
   d. Special attention to the baby—it's been a hard trip! Higher incidence of distressed infants at birth.
   e. Watch for increased risk of hemorrhage —massage the uterus firmly and regularly after placenta is out.

PROLONGED LABOR OR LACK OF PROGRESS

1. Lack of progress up to 2½ cm (latent phase) or even 4 cm is not of great concern. Latent phase can involve weak, irregular contractions with slow dilation and effacement and will still usually lead to strong, active labor. It is the longest phase of labor—important to get adequate rest and keep fluids up.

2. Slow progress poses no danger to the baby per se.[4] No progress can cause fetal distress and/or uterine rupture if contractions are strong.

3. Important in a long labor: monitor the fetal heart tones closely; make sure the mother is doing all right; make sure there is progress.

4. Possible causes of lack of progress:
   a. Uterine inertia (contractions weak and ineffectual). Can be caused by exhaustion.
   b. Disfunctional labor (irregular contractions, or contractions that seem strong but don't dilate the cervix).
   c. Atonic uterus (overstretched through twins or polyhydramnios).
   d. Malpresentation:
      (1) Breech often doesn't dilate the cervix as well.
      (2) Posterior position of the baby (baby's back of head against mother's back) is more uncomfortable; may take longer to rotate spontaneously and dilate cervix fully, may need to be turned by forceps, or may be born "sunnyside up."
   e. Undiagnosed cephalo-pelvic disproportion: suspect if the baby stays high and doesn't engage; lack of progress because the head is not pushing tightly against the cervix.
   f. Psychological factors: expectation, anxiety, inhibition. Check if anyone present is upsetting the mother. Check the energy of the room and send extra people away. Have her rest or get up and busy herself with something else. Talk through anything anyone is feeling (see Chapter 9).

5. When to go to the hospital:
   a. If the mother is exhausted, the baby's heart rate drops, the attendant is confused, or either parent has an intuition they should go to the hospital, go immediately.
   b. With a prolonged labor, the risk of postpartum hemorrhage rises (your attendant may have ergotrate or methergin to handle this).
   c. The average length of labor from 789 births managed by the Farm midwives was about 11 hours for first-time mothers and 7 hours for second or subsequent babies. The British Perinatal Study regards 24 hours as the outside limit for first stage. There are no hard-and-fast rules. Don't get trapped by your expectations. Keep assessing how the mother is, how the baby is, and if there is progress, even though slow. Also, remember that a long latent phase does not mean a

---

[4]Friedman's studies involving 3000 deliveries showed no increase in the infant death rate when there was a long early labor, long active labor, or long pushing stage (if forceps were not used). However, when dilation or descent had actually stopped, the infant death rate increased 16 times, even when forceps were not used. From Lewis Mehl, "Management of the Complication of Home Delivery: An Analysis of Results from the Santa Cruz Birth Center, California" in *Childbirth at Home* by Marion Sousa (New Jersey: Prentice-Hall, 1976) pp. 189-190.

great deal—91 percent of such labors will pick up and go into a successful delivery.[5]

   d. The point at which a mother experiencing a long labor should be taken to the hospital is very difficult to decide. The decision hinges on the birth attendant's confidence and competence, the energy reserves and intuition of the mother, and the continued well-being of the baby.

6. What is done at the hospital: sometimes nothing, sometimes a lot. Tools which the hospital has: IV solution for exhaustion, medication for postpartum hemorrhage, pitocin to strengthen failing contractions, forceps for rotation and extraction, pain medication, cesarean birth.

COMPLICATIONS OF SECOND STAGE (DESCENT AND BIRTH OF THE BABY)

LACK OF PROGRESS

1. Definition: Prolonged second stage is usually defined as more than two hours. Friedman[6] and Cohen[7] have both shown that a prolonged second stage in which there is slow descent of the head does not increase the risk to the baby born naturally (without forceps). Friedman found that any poor results encountered related to operative procedures such as forceps. Cohen found no increase in hemorrhage or postpartum infection in mothers who had a long second stage (even over three hours) and delivered without forceps or c-section.

2. Possible causes:
   a. Malpresentation (persistent posterior or head not completely flexed.)
   b. Head stuck in rotation to anterior position (transverse arrest).
   c. Variation in size of the pelvic cavity.
   d. Lack of adequate contractions (exhaustion).
   e. Head too large (undiagnosed cephalo-pelvic disproportion).
   f. Compound presentation (hand up beside the face).

3. What to do: If the cervix is fully dilated and the baby is not coming down the birth canal, try pushing with contractions. Also squat. This increases the size of the pelvis and the birth canal and lets gravity work with you.

4. When to go to the hospital:
   a. If there is fetal distress (monitor heart tones every 10 minutes in second stage, and after every contraction after two hours of pushing). However, if the birth is imminent, the attendant may do an episiotomy (or the woman may squat) to bring the baby out as quickly as possible; resuscitate if necessary.
   b. If the mother is exhausted or feels she wants to go to the hospital. Don't let pushing go on much over two hours if the labor has been particularly long and exhausting.
   c. If there is no progress after two hours of hard pushing (or if contractions aren't at all strong).

5. Hospital procedures:
   a. Low forceps or vacuum extraction are used if the baby is about to be born.
   b. Mid-forceps can be used (with spinal anesthesia) if the baby is about halfway down the birth canal; many hospitals would prefer a cesarean.
   c. A cesarean is preferred to high forceps if the baby isn't in the canal at all.
   d. Pitocin might be given if contractions have become weak.

FETAL DISTRESS DURING SECOND STAGE

1. If heart tones are around 110 or above 160, lie on your left side and recheck them; go to hospital if they don't pick up. If the birth is imminent, see 4a, above.

ARM, LEG OR BUTTOCKS COMING FIRST

1. An arm appearing first.
   a. May be a compound presentation (arm alongside of head). Should go to hospital, as delivery may be difficult with excessive tearing.

2. A leg or the buttocks presenting.
   a. Indicates an undiagnosed breech.
   b. If at all possible, GET TO THE HOSPITAL, as there is increased danger to the baby. Don't try to deliver a breech at home unless your attendant has good experience delivering breeches and good backup.
   c. If the baby is coming too fast, refer to the section on emergency undiagnosed breech delivery on p. 122.

BABY BORN IN THE MEMBRANES

1. If the baby is born with the "caul" over the face, make a hole in the membranes and remove from

---

[5]Emanuel A. Friedman, "An Objective Method of Evaluating Labor," *Hospital Practice*, July 1970.

   [6]Quoted by Lewis Mehl, *loc. cit.*

   [7]Wyane R. Cohen, "Influence of the Duration of Second Stage on Perinatal Outcome and Puerperal Morbidity," *Obstetrics and Gynecology*, Vol. 49, No. 3, March 1977, pp. 266–269.

face so he can start to breathe. (Folklore says this is good luck, and that the baby will never die by drowning.)

BABY'S HEAD IS OUT, CORD AROUND THE NECK

1. Incidence: about 30 percent of all births; usually presents no problem.

2. Feel all around the neck for the cord. Try bringing it up over the baby's head now or over the head or shoulders as the shoulders come out to prevent constricting the baby's throat or pulling on the placenta should the cord be short.

3. If the cord is around the neck twice and you are unable to loop it over the head, it should be clamped in two places and cut, as it may not have enough slack for the baby to be born without pulling on the placenta. Have the mother push, even without a contraction; the baby may need help starting to breathe.

4. If the cord is so tight that you can't get any slack up and the baby's head is becoming dark and congested, clamp or tie the cord in two places, cut, and urge the mother to push even before the next contraction. Be prepared to resuscitate the baby if necessary. Once the cord is cut, the baby's oxygen supply is cut off, so it shouldn't be cut unless it is too tight or impeding the baby's descent.

SHOULDERS DON'T COME OUT WITH THE NEXT CONTRACTIONS

1. The first shoulder is usually born with the next contraction. If not, watch for the head turning purple and encourage her to push. If they are still not born, the shoulders may be stuck on the pubic bone.

2. Incidence: 0.15 percent of all births.

3. Getting the mother into a squat or on hands and knees can open the pelvis and dislodge the top shoulder (Figure 8-5a).

4. Otherwise, you can hook your finger under the baby's lower arm and rotate it toward the baby's face, pulling gently outward. This will often rotate the baby slightly and release the upper shoulder from under the pubic bone (Figure 8-5b).

BABY BLUE AND NOT BREATHING, OR BORN WHITE AND LIMP

1. If you are just reading the manual, refer to "Breathing and Asphyxia in the Newborn" on p.

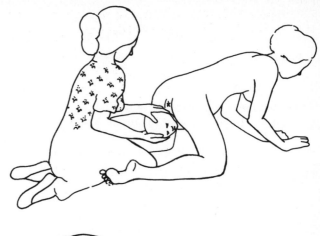

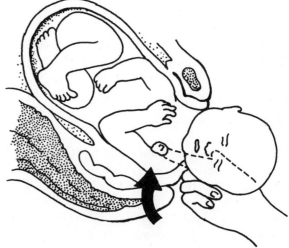

FIGURE 8-5. *(a) Hands and knees position for stuck shoulders. (b) "Corkscrew motion" to get the baby out.*

120 and "Cardio/pulmonary Resuscitation" on p. 121. Practice CPR now; attend the course given by your local Red Cross.

2. Baby in distress: blue or purple and not breathing.
   a. Keep warm, suction mouth and nose, stimulate body through touch, and the baby will start to gasp again of its own accord within the next minute or two.
   b. If breathing doesn't catch or you feel the baby needs it, do mouth-to-mouth resuscitation using only two cheeks full of air with each puff into baby's nose and mouth until it makes its own efforts to breathe.
   c. Don't cut the cord right away, as any oxygenated blood the baby is getting can help greatly.
   d. Don't use adult oxygen or release free-flowing oxygen near an infant due to the danger to its eyes if it is premature. Just do mouth-to-mouth until the baby responds with its own gasping.
   e. Once the baby's condition has stabilized, have

him checked by pediatrician or hospital. Be especially alert to the baby if he has been in distress. If the baby doesn't breathe and becomes white and limp, do CPR and transport to hospital immediately.

3. If the baby is born white and limp, it is in severe distress. It will not start to breathe again on its own, so you must take emergency measures:
   a. Suction nose and mouth, wrap to keep warm, put baby's head back slightly and give four quick puffs of air. Check for the heartbeat over the left nipple (whiteness indicates lack of circulation).
   b. If the heartbeat is missing, do cardiopulmonary resuscitation until the baby recovers or is transported to the hospital.
   c. If heartbeat is present, do mouth-to-mouth resuscitation using just two cheeks of air.

LOSS OF THE FETAL HEART TONES OR STILLBIRTH

1. If you don't feel the baby move for longer than 24 hours during pregnancy, check with your doctor. Failure to find the fetal heart tones is a sign of fetal death (other tests may be done). Your doctor will advise you about the onset or induction of labor. Losing a baby is always heartbreaking, and it can require special strength and support to carry and give birth to one that has died.

2. If you lose the heart tones during labor, don't panic. Feel how things are intuitively, and try again in a few minutes. Sometimes the baby moves, and there is a time during pushing when the pubic bone can make the heart tones extremely difficult to find.

3. If you still can't find the heart tones a few minutes later and feel the baby may have died, it's probably best to have a doctor check it out right away. You can then decide whether to go ahead and deliver in the hospital or to return home where you can deliver and grieve with your loved ones without interference.

4. If the baby is born and doesn't start to breathe, or if it comes out white and limp, do mouth-to-mouth or cardiopulmonary resuscitation right away (see preceding discussion, as well as p. 121).
   a. You'll have to decide whether you want to call the paramedics, take the baby to the hospital yourself while doing CPR, or stay at home until the baby revives or is dead. Whether at home or in the hospital, it is especially important in the grieving process that you hold the baby and be able to say goodbye to him or her.
   c. Then, by law, you must have a doctor come, or take the baby to the hospital, to have it pronounced dead and receive a death certificate.

COMPLICATIONS OF THIRD STAGE (AFTERBIRTH)

SHOCK WITH NO BLEEDING: CONCEALED HEMORRHAGE

1. Symptoms: Elevation in pulse of 10–15 beats/minute and drop in blood pressure of 15 mmHg in the diastolic reading may be first signs.
   a. Other signs include pallor, clamminess, chills, anxiety, eyes rolling back, etc.
   b. Refer to section on Shock on p. 113.
2. Cause: Probably bleeding behind a partially separated placenta.
3. EMERGENCY: GO TO HOSPITAL!
4. Usual treatment: manual removal of placenta under anesthesia and treatment for hemorrhage.

BLEEDING BEFORE DELIVERY OF THE PLACENTA

1. There should be one gush of blood as the placenta separates and another as she squats to deliver it. If it hasn't come out with squatting and she is continuing to bleed, you probably have hemorrhage with a partially separated placenta.
2. Elevate her legs and don't let her chill. Call ambulance and TRANSPORT TO HOSPITAL.
3. Usual treatment is manual removal under anesthesia and treatment for hemorrhage.

PLACENTA DOESN'T DELIVER WITHIN HALF HOUR

1. The placenta will usually separate within 20 to 30 minutes after the birth.
   a. Signs of separation include:
      (1) Lengthening of the cord.
      (2) Gush of blood.
      (3) Top of the uterus will rise.
      (4) Or uterus will become globular if placenta slips into birth canal.
      (5) Mother may feel a contraction.
   b. Get her up into a squat and have her push the placenta out (gravity helps).
2. Retained Placenta
   a. Definition: Placenta has separated but has not delivered within 30 minutes after the birth.

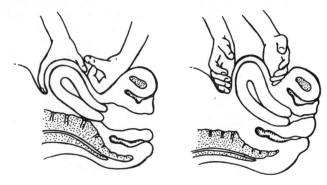

FIGURE 8-6. *Clamping the uterus for hemorrhage.*

    b. Cause: missing the separation when it occurred; difficulty is that the cervix may start to close down around it.

    c. What to do:

      (1) Squatting or sitting on the toilet; breastfeeding and nipple stimulation to bring on a contraction; angelica or blue cohosh tea (but be sure to urinate).

      (2) If your attendant is skilled at cord traction with uterine massage, it may deliver, but *do not* massage the uterus if the placenta is still attached (cause of hemorrhage).

    d. When to go to the hospital:

      (1) There is a lot of disagreement about how long you can wait for a placenta to deliver. The most important thing is that the mother's vital signs (including temperature) remain good and that the uterus feels firm so she isn't bleeding vaginally or behind the placenta (concealed hemorrhage).

      (2) If she is bleeding too much, call your paramedics and go to the hospital.

      (3) Even if vital signs are good, you should go to your doctor or emergency room if the placenta hasn't delivered within two hours.

    e. Treatment in the hospital: removal through cord traction, pitocin or manual removal if not separated.

3. Adherent Placenta

    a. Definition: When there are no signs that the placenta has left the upper uterine segment 30 minutes after birth: still attached to uterus.

    b. Usual cause: uterus not contracting and shrinking strongly enough to reduce the placental site and cause placenta to separate.

      (1) Contributing factors: anything which affects strength of contractions (exhausted uterus through precipitous delivery, overdistension, etc.) or affects the uterine lining (recent suction abortions, D & C's, recent previous pregnancy).

    c. What to do: stimulate contractions with breastfeeding, nipple stimulation, herbal teas as above. Do not massage the uterus.

    d. Danger of partial separation with concealed or gushing hemorrhage (more likely if uterus is massaged).

      (1) Call your paramedics and go to the hospital if there is bleeding or signs of shock; elevate the legs.

      (2) Manual removal is done under general anesthesia; hemorrhage is usually present.

PLACENTA INCOMPLETE WHEN EXAMINED

1. If the placenta appears to be missing a piece, (mother's side), uterus won't be able to contract and involute (shrink) properly.

    a. Likely to be excessive bleeding or delayed hemorrhage.

    b. Risk of infection is high.

2. If blood vessels don't stop before the edge (baby's side) there may be a separate lobe retained in the uterus. Danger as above.

3. If the membranes are missing or incomplete, they can cause infection.

4. What to do: Take the mother and placenta to the hospital to be examined. If incomplete, they will probably give pitocin or scrape the uterine lining under anesthesia.

EXCESSIVE BLEEDING ONCE PLACENTA IS OUT

1. Sign: Gushing hemorrhage or continual profuse bleeding.

2. Causes: Failure of the uterus to contract and close off the placental site, due to exhausted uterus (as with prolonged or precipitous delivery, multiparity), distended uterus (as with twins or polyhydramnios) or retained fragments of the placenta. Previous postpartum hemorrhage increases the probability this time, and anemia compounds the problem.

3. Unlikely to bleed to death, but NEEDS TO BE HANDLED quickly to stop blood loss:

4. What to do:

    a. If massaging the uterus doesn't stop blood loss, hold your hands clamped around the uterus (Figure 8-6). Keep it compressed for five minutes–longer if it starts to bleed again when you let up; all the way to the hospital if necessary.

    b. If not controlled, GO TO HOSPITAL.

    c. Elevate feet for shock.

    d. Re-examine placenta and take it with you.

5. Treatment: Doctors will usually give an IV with a drug such as pitocin to cause contraction of the uterus; may require plasma or blood transfusion.

CONSTANT TRICKLE OF BLOOD

1. Sign: She is bleeding too much if she is soaking two sanitary pads in a half hour.

2. Causes: Slow-trickle hemorrhage can be due to a retained fragment, a cervical tear, tearing of the birth canal or perineum.

3. Danger of fibrinogen anemia (loss of clotting factor) and bleeding to death.

4. MUST BE HANDLED. Go to hospital if necessary. Don't go to sleep without handling it.

TEARS OF THE PERINEUM AND BIRTH CANAL

1. Using sterile technique, examine the vulva, birth canal and labia for tears and decide whether they need stitches to heal well or not.

2. There are three degrees of severity in tearing:
   a. First degree—tearing of the skin just below or inside the vagina (Figure 8-7a).
   b. Second degree—tear extends into the perineum and its muscles (Figure 8-7b).
   c. Third degree—tear extends into the anal sphincter muscle (Figure 8-7c).

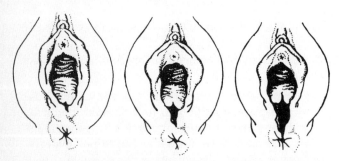

FIGURE 8-7. *(a) First-degree tear, (b) second-degree tear, and (c) third-degree tear.*

3. Stitching should be done within the first six hours after delivery to aid healing and decrease the risk of infection if stitched later.

BLEEDING AND DISCHARGE: POSTPARTUM

1. If in the hours after the birth you are soaking two sanitary pads in a half hour, bleeding is too heavy. See slow-trickle hemorrhage, above.

2. For the normal pattern of lochial discharge, see Chapter 11.

INFECTION

1. Sign: rise in temperature (100°F. or above), tenderness and pain in the abdomen, uterus enlarging, or foul-smelling discharge.

2. Postpartum infection can be serious, even leading to death from sepsis. SEE YOUR DOCTOR!

DEALING WITH MAJOR PROBLEMS

BREATHING AND ASPHYXIA IN THE NEWBORN

Babies really do start to breathe, and understanding the mechanism can help you to relax when the baby is normal and to act quickly when he or she is distressed. Once babies are born they will take several rapid, rhythmic gasps in an attempt to get oxygen.[8] If the baby succeeds in getting air into his lungs by this effort, he will continue to breathe, assuming he is otherwise healthy and not under anesthesia.

Primary Apnea

If, however, the baby does not succeed in expanding his lungs with these first gasping efforts, he will become apneic (*apnea* means a lack of breathing response). Such a baby would be characterized by:

1. a blue color, indicating adequate circulation of *un*oxygenated blood;
2. spontaneous activity or fairly good muscle tone;
3. heart rate usually above 100; and
4. reactivity, i.e., he will grimace when suctioned or will react when the attendant inserts a little finger into the baby's mouth and gently pulls the tongue forward.

The newborn in primary apnea will breathe again even if nothing is done, and there is no danger of brain damage during this period. Dr. Abramson points out that all of the "tricks" to stimulate breathing in newborns, such as spanking, jackknifing, alternating hot and cold water, etc., do not really accomplish anything because the baby will resume breathing efforts on his own; they are actually harmful to the infant and should never be used, he states.

This means that a baby who is not breathing, but is blue, shows fairly good muscle tone, and responds to stimulation, will start to breathe on his own (see Figure 8-8). There is a need for attentiveness, keeping the baby warm and suctioning the mouth and the nose (suctioning the nose first might cause the baby to swallow

---

[8]This section is based on David C. Abramson, M.D. "Delivery Room Management of the Distressed Infant," *American Family Physician*, Vol 6, No. 3, September 1972, pp. 60–68.

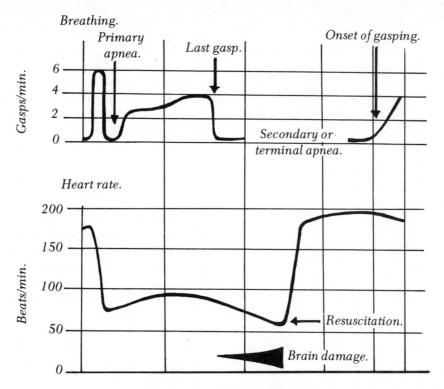

FIGURE 8-8. *Asphyxia in newborn.*

mucus in his throat). It is possible to wait patiently, rubbing the baby and watching for the next signs of breathing.

Secondary Apnea

After the period of primary apnea, the asphyxiated infant will begin to gasp again. If he is unable to aerate his lungs this time, he will again stop breathing and enter secondary or terminal apnea. A baby might be born in secondary apnea if he had experienced oxygen deprivation and tried to breathe while still inside his mother.

A baby in secondary apnea shows:

1. pallor, indicating failure of the circulation;

2. flaccidity or limpness, lack of muscle tone;

3. heart rate of less than 100; and

4. no response to forward pressure on the tongue (i.e., unreactive to stimuli).

The attendant can recognize this condition by the pallor and flaccidity of the baby's head and neck as they emerge.

Asphyxial brain damage begins about one minute after the onset of secondary apnea. No time should be wasted trying to stimulate breathing since all such efforts are doomed to failure. The only chance for successful resuscitation is getting oxygen into the infant's lungs by the quickest method familiar to the resuscitator.

If resuscitation equipment for the newborn is not available, mouth-to-mouth resuscitation should begin immediately, using two cheeks full of air (see next section on CPR). The heart rate should increase within 15 seconds after the start of adequate resuscitation in most newborns in secondary apnea. However, if the initial heart rate was less than 50, cardiac massage should also be done, according to Dr. Abramson. This should be maintained until the baby starts to breathe on its own.

THE NEWBORN IN DISTRESS: CARDIOPULMONARY RESUSCITATION (CPR)

If the baby is blue and his breathing efforts are not successful, it means his circulation is good and the baby just needs mouth-to-mouth resuscitation (Steps 1–4 following). If the baby is white and limp, do not wait for him to make his own efforts to breathe, as you have a severely distressed infant. Proceed with full CPR.

1. Suction the mouth, then the nose, with a sterile bulb syringe to remove mucus which may be blocking the air passage.

2. Put the baby over your arm (head in your palm, feet tucked under your arm) or on a hard surface and tilt the head back to make the airway straight (Figure 8-9). (Letting the head go back too far again occludes the air passage.)

3. You now have an *open airway*. If the baby is still

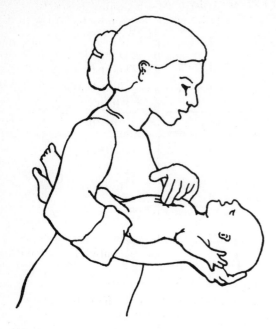

FIGURE 8-9.

not breathing, take two cheeks full of air and place your mouth over the baby's nose *and* mouth, creating a seal. Give a short puff into the baby, using only your cheeks (using your lungs can rupture the baby's lungs). If the lungs have not expanded, the first puff will need to expand them, but mustn't be hard enough to injure them. Give the baby four quick puffs of air.

4. Check for the baby's heartbeat by feeling over the left nipple with the first two fingers of your hand (practice on a baby or a young child now—the heartbeat in a normal newborn is 120–160). If you can't feel the heartbeat, continue with Step 5. If the heart is beating on its own, pressure on the chest might interfere with its rhythms and cause the baby to get worse. If the baby's circulation is good but he still isn't breathing (blue color, good or even fair heartbeat and some muscle tone), just do mouth-to-mouth resuscitation, delivering about one puff every 2½ seconds (24/minute).

5. If there is no heartbeat, apply pressure on the sternum just between the nipples with the first two fingers of your hand. Push the chest down about ½ inch, about 80–100 times a minute, which will circulate blood through the baby. It's quite rapid and needs to be in a steady rhythm.

6. Every fifth beat, *as you lift your fingers up,* blow two cheeks full of air into the baby's nose and mouth without interrupting your rhythm of pressing on the chest. Push five times, blow between pushes, push five times, blow. Keep up a steady rhythm until the baby starts to come round or until the baby reaches the hospital.

Practice this on a doll now. It takes a bit of practice to be able to maintain the steady rhythm on the chest. **Take the Red Cross Course on CPR.** It only takes two evenings of your time, and you can practice on the special doll in which the chest actually depresses and inflates. You also learn adult CPR. These are valuable skills for everyone to have, and well worth the investment. **CPR saves lives.**

EMERGENCY UNDIAGNOSED BREECH DELIVERY

Because of the increased risk to the baby, you should not attempt a breech delivery at home unless you have a birth attendant skilled in breech births and excellent emergency equipment and backup.

Dangers to the baby include a longer labor, since the head isn't dilating the cervix, and the possibility of the cervix clamping down around the head once the body has slipped out. Also, the head doesn't clear the pelvic cavity until the body is already born, so the head may get stuck on the bones if the baby is particularly large; the head also doesn't have the opportunity to mold as it does in a vertex presentation. And the cord becomes pinched between the head and the pelvis once the baby is born to the navel, so the baby may suffer from lack of oxygen. Prolapse of the cord is also more common since the buttocks often don't fit tightly into the pelvic cavity. Fractures, dislocations and nerve damage are more common with breech births, as is asphyxiation.

If you unexpectedly see or feel the buttocks or feet, get to the hospital, or have the mother squat. Delivering in a squatting position eliminates most of the problems discussed below. Let nature and gravity work and keep your hands off!

This is the classic method of delivering a breech, recommended before we had seen it done squatting.

1. Meconium staining is common because of the position and is not a sign of distress per se.

2. Never pull on the baby or try to free the legs until the body is born to the navel.

3. Have the mother push as hard as she can with contractions, and have someone keep manual pressure on her belly in the direction that the baby is coming out to help with the delivery and to help keep the baby's head flexed (Figure 8-10).

4. Once the navel is showing, pull down a loop of cord so there is no strain on the baby's navel (Figure 8-11). The pulse in the cord should be strong.

5. Have someone call out one-minute intervals from the time the cord is showing. Everyone should stay calm and remember to breathe.

    Once the cord is visible, it is being compressed between the baby and the mother's pelvis, which

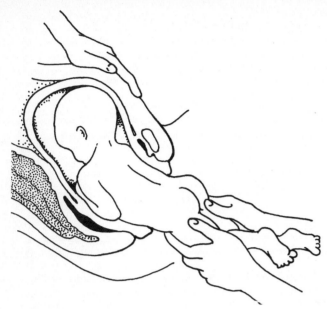

FIGURE 8-10. *Breech birth: manual pressure with hands supporting.*

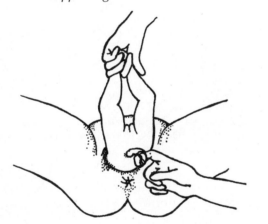

FIGURE 8-11. *Breech birth: Pulling down a loop of cord.*

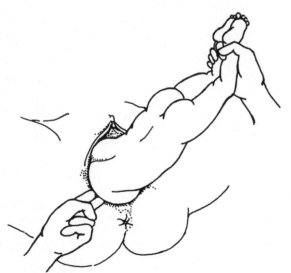

FIGURE 8-12. *Breech birth: Freeing the arms, if necessary.*

cuts off the baby's oxygen supply. The baby needs to be born within eight or ten minutes or it will die of suffocation. If the baby isn't born within five or six minutes, gentle, calm help may be given. (Gregory White, M.D., states that more breech babies die of injuries received at the hands of their would-be rescuers than die of suffocation.[9])

6. If the birth from the navel to the armpit is not accomplished with the next contraction, gentle pulling on the legs might be helpful, *keeping the baby's back towards the mother's stomach* (the baby's back should never turn toward the mother's back).

7. The arms are usually on the baby's chest. They need to come out before the head. Wearing a sterile glove, run your fingers up the baby's back, over the shoulder and down the chest, sweeping the baby's arm down across the chest with it. Do this with the bottom shoulder, then lower the baby and repeat with the top shoulder (Figure 8-12).

    If an arm is stuck over the head, it is necessary to bring it down across the chest. If stuck behind the neck, rotate the baby's body in the direction the hand is pointing until the arm is freed.

8. Wrap the body in a receiving blanket to prevent chilling and inhibiting the breathing response.

9. Keep the baby's back toward the mother's belly. Lower the body until you see the nape of the neck and the hair, then raise the body so that the face sweeps the perineum (Figure 8-13).

10. Suction the baby's airways as soon as the head is out. Maintain perineal support so the rest of the head is born as slowly as possible (too rapid a change in pressure can be damaging to the baby).

    If the baby's head is stuck, put your arm under his body with your middle finger in the baby's mouth and your ring and index fingers on each side of the baby's cheekbones. The purpose is to keep the baby's head flexed, *not to pull the baby out.* With your other hand (or an assistant's), push on the mother's abdomen (Figure 8-14).

    If the head does not come, don't pull, since you might permanently injure the baby's spinal cord or the nerves of his arms and breathing mechanism. If the head cannot be delivered without undue force, maintain an air passage to the baby's nose by pressing the vaginal walls away from the baby's nose and mouth until a doctor arrives to complete the delivery (Figure 8-15).

    Dr. White emphasizes that more damage is done by someone exercising too much force than by

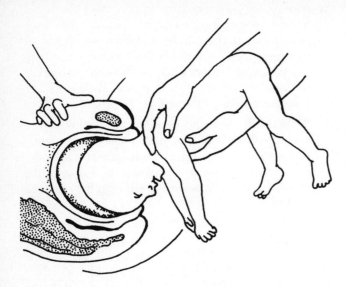

FIGURE 8-13. *Breech birth: The gentle birth of the head.*

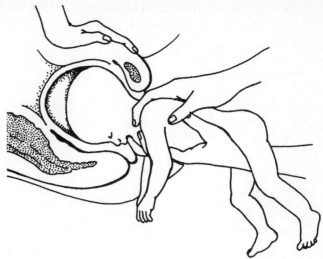

FIGURE 8-14. *Breech birth: Keeping head flexed, if necessary, by inserting a finger in the baby's mouth.*

breeches being stuck. He ends his section on breech birth by teaching you how to baptize, so take care (see "Matthew's birth" on p. 128).

UNDIAGNOSED TWINS

Twins should not be attempted at home without attendants who are skilled in the birth of twins and good emergency backup in case of complications. The second twin is breech in about 50 percent of cases, and the babies often require intensive care (Figure 8-16).

1. The cord is always clamped in two places just in case there are undiagnosed twins. Otherwise, the second twin could bleed to death if they share a common circulation.

2. You may suspect an undiagnosed twin if the top of your uterus is way above your umbilicus once your baby is out (or when the second baby starts to be born!).

3. With a long sterile glove, feel vaginally to see what position the second twin is in. It should be born within 15 to 20 minutes. If you have time you might go to the hospital or call for medical assistance, especially if it is not head down.

4. If the spontaneous delivery of the second twin does not occur within twenty minutes, you should go to the hospital. They may need to rotate the baby internally; the mother may require pitocin to get good strong contractions.

5. The placenta or placentas deliver after both babies are born. There is more likely to be problems with separation since it covers a larger area of the uterus.

6. Postpartum hemorrhage is also more common

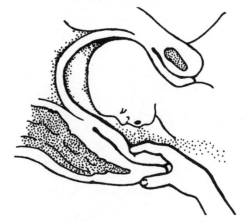

FIGURE 8-15. *Breech birth: Maintaining an air passage for the baby.*

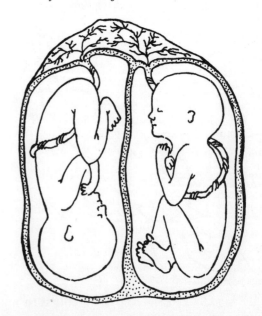

FIGURE 8-16. *A common presentation for twins.*

because of the large placental site and the overextension of the uterus, causing a lack of tone so it doesn't clamp down as well.

7. The second twin tends to have more problems than the first, and the probability of problems increases the longer his birth is delayed. Both babies should be suctioned and watched closely for respiratory problems and kept warm. They should be weighed, and should be seen by a pediatrician as soon as possible.

IF YOU NEED TO GO TO THE HOSPITAL

Parents who are going to have a baby at a birth center or hospital sometimes want to know how to keep it spiritual. You can do that by just having a good time and visibly enjoying your baby. In hospitals they see this so infrequently that most nurses love it, and they'll probably come in and want to hang out with you. Sometimes, look at a nurse you feel good with—look in her eyes during a rush. It's obvious that if a husband loves his wife and is able to give her good support, it can make a material difference of several hours of labor and make a difference between pain and ecstasy.*

If something comes up and you need to go to the hospital during labor, remember that you are still you, and you can still have a positive birth experience. You and your partner create your own environment, and whether in a hospital or at home, you can still maintain the psychic awareness which affirms birth and is in touch with the being of your baby.

Keep Your Intention

If you are going to the hospital, it is because some specific signs or events have occurred. You haven't "failed" at having a homebirth—rather, you are going to the specialists for some variation from normal labor—which is why hospitals exist. There is no right or wrong way to have a baby, and although you may feel disappointed or apprehensive, concentrate on your breathing and look forward to meeting your baby.

If you have a private doctor who has agreed to meet you at the hospital, you are already familiar with him and his procedures. If you have to go to the emergency room, you may experience flak from any doctors or nurses who are opposed to homebirth and see you as having done something wrong. This is not what you need to hear in a moment of uncertainty, but realize that it is their misdirected way of expressing concern for you and your baby, and let their words flow by. Get down to the business at hand!

*Ina May Gaskin, quoted in *Practicing Midwife*, Vol. 1, No. 5, p. 5.

Medical Procedures

Some of the medical procedures which you are likely to encounter (depending on where you are in labor and the nature of the complication) include the following.

Admission Paper work, checking dilation, blood pressure, temperature, shaving the pubic hair (ask for a "mini clip" if possible), an IV drip of glucose to combat fatigue and keep your fluid level up and to have a vein already open for administering drugs or replacing blood.

Electronic Fetal Monitor The external monitor consists of two belts which go around your belly and are connected by wires to a machine which amplifies the baby's heartbeat as well as giving a printout (like a ticker tape) showing the strength and duration of uterine contractions. An internal monitor is often used once the waters have broken because it is more accurate. A thin tube is inserted between the uterus and the baby's head to measure the strength of contractions (it is then strapped to your leg), and an electrode is fastened to the baby's scalp to monitor the heartbeat.

Pitocin If labor has stopped, or if contractions are weak and irregular, you may be given pitocin, which is the name for synthetic oxytocin, the hormone in your body which causes uterine contractions. It is usually given intravenously through the IV drip. Depending on the dosage given, contractions may feel different and be harder to handle, or may be much like a normal labor.

Rupturing the Membranes This is often done to speed up labor. While not to be advocated as a routine procedure, it can help with lack of progress. Contractions are usually stronger once the waters break, and are especially strong if you are receiving pitocin (check what the IV bottle says on it). You may need direct coaching.

Anesthesia If you are being offered a spinal just to make you more comfortable, feel free to decline. But if they are going to rotate the baby's head or deliver him with forceps, a regional anesthetic may be necessary. It is usually given to you in the delivery room. You lie on your side, rounding your back. An area on the lower back is numbed and the anesthetic is put into your spinal column either in a single injection or by a continuous drip through a catheter. The most common types are spinal, saddle block, continuous caudal, and epidural.

If you have a choice, the epidural seems to allow the most sensation (they all immobilize you from the waist down) so you are able to help a bit more with pushing, and it has the least side effects since it doesn't penetrate the spinal fluid. If you do have a spinal rather than an epidural, don't raise your head up suddenly, and stay flat for about eight hours to avoid the spinal headache which is often an aftereffect.

A pudendal bloc injected vaginally into your

pudendal nerve may be all that is required for low forceps.

Cesarean Unless you are involved in a time-pinch emergency, you can ask for a second opinion about the necessity of the operation. If time is of the essence, you may be given a general anesthetic, which takes effect more rapidly, but leaves you totally unconscious. Otherwise, you can request a regional anesthetic which allows you to relate with your baby immediately after it is born and leaves you less groggy. Some hospitals are beginning to allow the father to be present, so request it. A curtain is put up so you don't see the incision. *Ask that the cut be horizontal, rather than the classical vertical incision.* You shouldn't feel any pain, but may feel a great deal of pulling.

More and more hospitals are moving toward making the cesarean birth experience as positive and family-centered as possible, so ask to have the baby in the operating room to hold or even to nurse. Also, cesarean support groups such as C/SEC may have chapters in your area which can help you after the birth.

Many hospitals have rooming-in, so the baby can be with you most or all of the time and you can nurse as usual. Friends who have had a cesarean birth say that the most painful part is afterwards and advise against refusing painkillers so you have energy for your baby (rather than exhausting yourself, coping with the pain.) The best pick-me-up for a tired mom is to have the baby with her; separation just increases the desire to be apart, whereas the more a mother is with her baby, the more she wants it. As a cesarean mother, you can probably expect a hospital stay of from three to five days, and when you go home realize that you are going to be recovering from surgery as well as having a new baby, so make sure to get extra help. Don't be surprised if your emotions are really volatile, and talk with your partner and others about how you are feeling.

No longer is it necessary to have an automatic repeat cesarean. Support for having a vaginal birth after a cesarean (VBAC) continues to grow, but you still may have trouble finding a truly supportive doctor or midwife. *Silent Knife* by Cohen and Estner and organizations such as C/SEC and the Cesarean Prevention Movement have been instrumental in helping women know that this option is possible for them. *Silent Knife* offers invaluable help for resolving feelings about a cesarean birth and ways to find support for a VBAC. Many women who had a cesarean for "cephalopelvic disproportion" have given birth vaginally to even larger babies the next time.

Requests for the Baby

If you end up delivering in the hospital, there are certain things you can ask about:

- Request the LeBoyer bath—many hospitals allow it at the discretion of the doctor.
- Request Ilotycin instead of silver nitrate for the baby's eyes (it burns less), and request that the drops not be put in immediately.
- Ask to hold and nurse the baby on the delivery table.
- Request an early visit by the pediatrician, which is necessary if you want to leave early.
- If you and the baby are both doing fine, you can leave the hospital whenever you want, as early as a few hours after delivery. You may have to sign yourself out "against medical advice" for their insurance purposes, but it is an option open to you if there are no complications.
- If you do stay in the hospital, insist on rooming-in, so that your baby stays in your room instead of in the nursery. This helps with breastfeeding and lets you love your baby without schedules.
- Ask that it be written on your baby's record that you are breastfeeding, that he not be given formula or sugar water, and that he be brought to you on demand if you aren't able to get rooming-in.

IF YOU MUST TAKE YOUR BABY TO THE HOSPITAL

Don't lose your awareness that your baby is a being, and you don't need to hand him or her over to the hospital like a small bundle—you can keep informing yourselves and keep participating in the decision-making process. If you have already contacted a pediatrician who is aware of the importance of breastfeeding and of families being together, you are several steps ahead. Otherwise remember that you can always request a second opinion.

If your baby is yellow from jaundice, treat him at home with sunlight or fluorescent lights. If your doctor wants hospitalization, ask if you can't set up bili lights at home or stay with your baby in the hospital. (See Chapter 10).

If your baby is hospitalized for some birth defect or other complication (or if he is born prematurely in the hospital), try to spend as much time as possible with him, touching and holding him whenever you can, and breastfeeding as soon as possible. (Express your milk and take it to the hospital until then; La Leche League often has breast pumps they can lend you.)

If your baby is distressed at birth and comes around, pay close attention to his breathing, skin color, eye contact and sucking reflex. If they are strong, the damage probably hasn't been too great and you might want to hold and nurse the baby and give him a chance to recuperate and find his own rhythms before having him checked by a doctor or hospital. When babies come into the hospital after distress or trauma, they are often taken away from the parents and subjected to enough tests and electronic gadgetry, in my opinion, to put anyone into shock. However, if your baby's vital signs are not good or if he shows any of the danger signs in the newborn (Chapter 10), you shouldn't delay in seeing a pediatrician.

If your baby is in serious condition and needs immediate emergency care and you have no pediatrician lined up, call your paramedics and tell them you will need neonatal intensive care. Some ambulances are especially equipped for transporting newborns. You will probably be feeling very emotional and lost at the hospital, not knowing what is happening with your baby. And when you see him again he may be hooked up to several life-support machines. It can be very emotionally draining to have a premature baby or one with problems, but don't fail to touch and love him for fear of loss. Prayer and wanting him to live may be the factor that tips the scales.

But babies are amazingly hearty and can withstand things such as oxygen deprivation much better than a child or adult. They withstand the traumas not only of birth but of modern medicine very well. If you do require anesthesia, forceps or a cesarean delivery, don't burden yourself with added worry about the effects on the baby; the chances are that he'll come through at least as well as most of us did from our births. If your baby's birth becomes one requiring expert medical technology for a safe outcome, be grateful that we live in a time and place where it is available to us.

IF YOUR BABY DIES

No one who is pregnant wants to contemplate the possibility of her baby's dying, but many of us are coming to feel that reclaiming our lives from mechanization and unconsciousness has to include acknowledging and looking at death—indeed, *rehumanizing* it. After all, none of us will escape experiencing the death of loved ones at some point in our lives or the lives of those close to us.

If your baby is born dead or dies at home, see the section on stillbirth (p. 118) for things you need to do. If he dies in a hospital, you have the right to see and hold the baby, to be alone with him to say goodbye. This can be important in helping you come to terms with his death. You also have the right to make your own arrangements for burial.

No matter under what circumstances someone dies, those remaining think, "If only I had . . ." This is a normal part of the grieving cycle, and it is important neither to deny nor to feed any feelings of grief, guilt, anger, or frustration that you will probably go through, so that you can come to acceptance and go on.

The pain of death can only heal with time. Don't be afraid to feel the love and the grief, for they are part of being human and unite us with all other people.

We especially recommend you read the book *Ended Beginnings* by Claudia Panuthos for much-deserved help.

KEEPING THINGS IN PERSPECTIVE

Having detailed the possible complications, let me emphatically reaffirm that birth is a normal physiological process for which your body is well-suited, and that 90–95 percent of prepared homebirths proceed without any problem. However, you may have come to see why many doctors, who spend 95 percent of their time studying complications and may rarely see a normal birth, [10] are so reluctant to let anyone deliver without the technological equipment they were trained to use.

What I have tried to provide in this chapter is as complete a guide as possible for homebirth parents, so that if you are among the small percentage of women who develop a problem during labor or delivery, you will know what is happening and have a positive experience (see the two birth accounts following).

In this chapter, I have described emergency backup in terms of the Western medical system because that is the most familiar and the most accessible to us. But I recognize that it is only one approach to the body and the spirit. For example, if we were acupuncturists, we would monitor the woman's pulses instead of taking her blood pressure and would stimulate labor and lessen discomfort through acupuncture points rather than through pitocin and anesthesia. We fall back on what we know when things are not normal. Let me urge you to fall back on common sense (and on prayer, if you pray), both before and during medical procedures.

Obviously you, like everyone else, are interested in a safe, joyous birth experience. That is one of the reasons you're planning a homebirth. As Chapter 1 shows, planned homebirths with prenatal care and skilled attendants are statistically as safe or safer than hospital births, while avoiding many of the complications induced by an overly medicalized approach. There are risks in homebirth. There are also risks in hospital birth. The decision, the "informed consent," must be yours.

I would hope that hospitals will someday give their patients as much information about the incidence of complications in their institutions as homebirth couples are coming to have about out-of-hospital birth. Every hospital should list their percentage of complications,

---

[10] A friend of mine who had recently become a doctor decided to go back and do a rotation in obstetrics because so many of his friends were having homebirths. He reported that out of 200 births at County General, not one could have been called "normal." He would have done better, in my opinion, to have worked with a homebirth doctor or a good midwife.

emergencies, deaths, standard procedures and costs, and not only make that information available to the public, but see that it is given to every pregnant couple planning to deliver there. Then in a given community there might be the possibility of real consumer choice and a revolution in birthing practices.

DEALING WITH EMOTIONS

Whenever something does not go the way you had planned, there can be disappointment and a sense of loss. Grieving can occur for something seemingly minor in a normal birth or for major complications involving a cesarean, stillbirth or birth defects. Several books have been written to help women with their emotions after a birth that had complications, and many communities have support groups as well.

FOR FURTHER READING

Emergency Childbirth by Dr. Gregory White. Clearly written for nonmedical attendants. Recommended for parents.

Ended Beginnings by Claudia Panuthos and Catherine Romeo. A healing book for all types of childbearing loss.

Heart and Hands: A Midwifes Guide, by Elizabeth Davis. Extremely clear and well-written. Very understandable.

Midwifery by Jean Hallum. A simple and concise text, understandable by parents.

For detailed work with psychological aspects, see *Pregnant Feelings* by Rahima Baldwin and Terra Palmarini, *Transformation Through Birth* by Claudia Panuthos, and *Silent Knife* by Cohen and Estner.

AN UNEXPECTED BREECH: THE BIRTH OF MATTHEW KENNA

Rick and Wendy Kenna hadn't been able to find a birth attendant and were determined to do a homebirth themselves. A friend of theirs who was a nurse recommended they attend my homebirth classes, so they drove the two hours each way to attend weekly classes. This is the letter I received from them after the birth.

Dear Rahima,

Have been meaning to sit down and write to you sooner, but between having a new baby and moving, I've been very busy. Just wanted to let you know how our birth went. I went into labor at 4:30 A.M. I had had false labor twice, so I wasn't really sure if it was the real thing. But at about 8:30 the mucous plug came out and the contractions began to get stronger. I was really happy to have learned the breathing and relaxation as this helped me to remain calm and in control. Rick never left my side, and I don't think I could have handled it without him.

By 4:30 P.M. the water broke and I was almost through transition. At 6:00 nothing much was happening. I wasn't having any urge to push, although my body seemed to be pushing. The contractions weren't much different than transition contractions. Then Rick noticed something in the birth canal. He thought it was the cord coming down ahead of the baby. It was blue and looked twisted. We didn't have any birth attendant, just Rick, but some friends had come to take us to the hospital if the need should arise. So they carried me to

the car and rushed me to the hospital in a knee-chest position.

When we got to the hospital (it was about a three-minute drive) I was examined. What Rick had seen was not the cord, but three little blue toes! The baby was breech. My doctor seemed to think the baby turned the last few days, but I feel he was breech all along because I could feel the same little round spot I had always felt.

Matthew wasn't born until 10:32 P.M. My contractions were very weak. If I would make myself push at the start of the contraction, the urge to push would overtake me. The doctors and hospital were very cooperative. They didn't force any routine hospital procedures on us. We remained in control of the situation, which was nice.

They did have to take his head with forceps, though, because the cervix started to close around it. He inhaled while still inside me, so they had to suction him pretty thoroughly. He was a beautiful baby—about 6 lbs. 10 oz., and 20½ inches long. By one-month-old he was 8 lbs. 6 oz. and had grown an inch. He's a calm baby, very good.

We both regretted having to go to the hospital, but we're happy our baby is alive. He probably would have died at home. I wish I had drunk more liquids, as I got very tired during pushing. For me, the pushing was much harder than transition.

My original reason for wanting to have the baby at home was because I was disgusted with doctors and hospitals. After going through labor at home, my reasons for wanting to have a baby at home are much different. It was so much easier to stay relaxed and calm. We plan to try it at home again next time.

We are very thankful for the things we learned in your classes. It was one of the best investments we made.

Sincerely,
Wendy, Rick and Matthew Kenna

THE BIRTH OF MAGNUS BY CESAREAN SECTION

Dianne and Marc Schevene

Dianne:

When I became pregnant, there was no doubt that I wanted this baby to be born at home. We had waited years for this child and I had read and learned a lot. I felt well-prepared by the Informed Homebirth classes and was confident that we would have a very positive experience. No amount of imagining could let me know in advance how the birth would go, so I kept reminding myself the most important thing is to stay in the present and flow with whatever happens.

I started labor around 4:00 A.M., so I got up and cleaned house, which was my way of making final preparations and dealing with the rushes of excitement. Timing contractions gave me something to do and I went overboard, timing almost every contraction all morning. From nine to ten o'clock contractions were three minutes apart and I hoped the birth wouldn't happen before our friends arrived from Boulder. I wanted to have their support and share this with them.

The day was really mellow. I was happy and occupied with the work at hand.

Allison, an obstetrical nurse, Rahima and her family arrived in late afternoon from Boulder, several hours away. Our two friends from Breckenridge, John and Carol, were already there. I really slowed down, as if I had forgotten what was happening. Then things picked up and I went in the room Marc had prepared for the birthing. From then on I lost track of time. I just kept breathing and resting.

Dilation was checked and thought to be 6 cm, but my uterus was tipped way off to the right and it was hard to feel my whole cervix. I was real excited that things had gone so smoothly and figured we'd have a baby before much longer. Friends took turns massaging me and when Marc took off his shirt and lay next to me, I felt wonderful.

Later they checked me again and there had been no change in dilation, but my uterus had straightened out. Having a baby was getting to be hard work. I began to

feel a little tired and discouraged, but didn't have time to think about it because I had my work to do.

After several hours more, dilation remained the same. As my labor seemed to fizzle, so did I. We decided to call the doctor about 2:00 A.M. At the clinic he said I was actually only 4 cm dilated, and I really felt let down. Things certainly weren't progressing and we decided to head for the hospital about fifty miles away.

The ride was a relaxing change for me. I was glad we had open communication with our doctor and that we had no qualms about going to the hospital when the situation called for it.

When I got situated in the labor bed, I cried from tiredness and discouragement, knowing what might lie ahead. The admitting nurse came in and said she was sorry. I said that I wasn't ashamed to be human. I felt in touch with what was happening. I was really glad we had been so prepared for this birth. I knew what was going on and that kept me from being afraid.

Our doctor broke the waters to see if it would do anything and had the nurse set up an IV. She had wanted the night off. I was angry with her for taking so long to put in an IV; I'd been in labor over 23 hours and she was just prolonging everything. I stayed at 4 cm, so they started a pitocin drip and gradually increased it. The baby's heartbeat was strong and it was reassuring to hear it broadcast over the monitor.

When the shifts changed a nurse came in who was rather unpleasant. She accepted Marc but was annoyed that Allison and Rahima were still with me. When she left the room, I asked my doctor if she had to be there. He must have said something to her, because from then on she was terrific.

My contractions still didn't become regular, though I had more discomfort, and I began to realize that no progress would be made. I wanted to get on with it and asked the doctor how long before he would check me again. He said, "Fifteen minutes." I thought, "I can't do this fifteen more minutes." And then I thought,

"You've been doing it for twenty-four hours, you can do it fifteen more minutes!"

The decision was made to go ahead with a cesarean. That was the lowest moment: tears mixed with tiredness and relief. I knew my baby would be born soon and I could rest. When the pitocin was stopped and the monitor taken off, it was a lot easier to handle contractions.

We learned a lot about c-sections really fast. There wasn't anyone available to do a spinal. In a section with total anesthesia it's essential to get the baby out before any drugs reach it, so all the prepping was done while I was awake, most of it in the labor room. I was reassured to hear the doctor and nurses talking about how fast the surgeon was.

The anesthetist came and explained what she would use and how it would affect me. She'd had two cesarean births and was very reassuring. The nurse who prepped me, including shaving my abdomen and inserting a catheter, always told me what she was doing. I answered some questions, and Marc and I signed a paper. Marc and I said good-bye as I was wheeled into the operating room. Allison was allowed to be there. She coached me through the last few contractions while final prepping was done. I was draped and there was a drape between my head and body. EKG wires were attached to my chest and my abdomen was scrubbed. In between contractions I could feel my baby fluttering and kicking, letting me know everything was okay right up until I was unconscious. I heard the word "Ready" and I was out. Our son was born within one and one-half minutes.

The next thing I can recall is being in recovery feeling groggy, chewing on a washcloth, hurting, and seeing Marc holding a white bundle. I asked if it was our baby and found out we had a son. I was ecstatic. Marc asked if I wanted to hold him, but I didn't think I could manage that. He held Magnus next to my face and I saw and touched him for the first time. Later I heard that Magnus' Apgars were 9 and 10, so he obviously hadn't been drugged. Also, learning that Marc had been with him and cared for him when I couldn't, right after the birth, made me feel warm and happy all over.

In my room, they put Magnus in an isolette next to my bed so whenever I was alert I could see him. As soon as I was conscious I asked to have him in bed with me and there he stayed most of the time until we went home.

They had me up and walking the first evening after he ws born. I was still on IV's, so one nurse walked me and one walked the bottles. Since I'd been lying down all day, a lot of blood had accumulated, and when I stood up I gushed. It concerned me at first, but the nurses assured me it was normal.

I was recovering from childbirth just as anyone would, bleeding a bit and having to massage my uterus so it would go down, and I was also recovering from surgery. I felt great joy to have Magnus with me, and I hurt from surgery. The pain didn't diminish the joy nor did the joy lessen the pain. I think caring for Magnus kept my mind off the discomfort and helped me recover quickly. I just wanted to take my baby home.

I was given shots for pain when I asked, and I decided not to be stoic about it because I needed to rest and have the energy to be with Magnus. I arranged everything so I could change him and care for him myself right in bed. It felt so good to touch him and take care of him myself. The second night I was really tired, so I decided he should sleep in his bassinet and I had some help caring for him.

I got to like the nurses a lot. They were great helping me to get started breastfeeding. I was very dry and Magnus lost 10 ounces the second day. Blood tests were done. I felt helpless and worried. I missed Marc terribly. I had a good cry which relieved a lot of tension. The doctor said to give him glucose water because his blood sugar was low and he was beginning to dehydrate. I realized that my images of how things should go didn't matter at all. If sugar water was the best thing for him, it didn't matter what I'd read or thought ahead of time.

When Marc arrived I relaxed a lot. I decided I needed skin-to-skin contact with my new boy so I took off my hospital gown and stripped him to his diaper and held him next to me. I just touched him, looked at him and marveled with Marc. I thought that nine months might seem long enough to form an ear, but to think his whole body was made in that amount of time was outrageous.

The third day the dressings were removed. My abdomen was still very large, and seeing the incision for the first time blew all my fantasies about what my body would look like after having the baby. I got to take a bath, and the relaxation helped relieve a lot of tension and pain.

I had a postoperative fever and I had to drink plenty of fluids for the next couple of weeks. I quit taking pain medication 36 hours after the operation, which helped recovery, but it took quite a while for the drugs to work out of my system. I had to cough to keep fluid from accumulating in my lungs. My intestines didn't start to function again for two days.

The fourth day my surgeon said I could go home. I was so excited! Driving home Marc and I shared our grateful feelings. I was glad to be alive and have our baby, thankful for the kind treatment we had received from our doctor and the hospital staff and for the support of our friends. We were fortunate to live in a time and place where modern medical techniques were available. Most of all we were happy to be sharing such a high experience.

(After the operation, her doctor said that the baby's head was way over to the side so the vertex wasn't pre-

senting, resulting in disproportion and lack of dilation.
Rahima)

Marc:
We had made arrangements to go to the hospital in case we had problems, but we really didn't know what to expect. And I felt frightened, sitting there in the waiting room not knowing what was going on, feeling very isolated, alone, scared. After all that training for a homebirth, here I sat feeling helpless. Waiting.

The previous twenty-five hours had been easy, even the decision to go to the hospital. Once we had decided to have our baby at home, the next step was to find out what to do, what not to do, and when to go to the hospital if necessary. With the knowledge that came mainly from the Homebirth class, but also from other readings and conversations, I felt confident that we were ready to have our baby at home. My job was really very simple. I had to recognize what was happening and either keep Dianne relaxed and let her know that everything was going fine, or else decide that something was happening that I didn't understand and call the doctor.

There were others there too: Rahima, Allison, Wahhab and John, but that day of waiting seemed to be just for Dianne and me, as if all the others were vague forms in the background. They were a tremendous help, of course, but my consciousness was only with Dianne.

I understood what was happening, I felt confident in my responsibility as decision maker, and I knew that I would be able to deliver the baby. At the same time I was both awestruck by what was happening and acutely aware. At that time I felt no fear; I knew what was happening. The time passed slowly, invisibly. There was little to do. No running around. John made sure we had gas in the car.

After twenty hours, dilation had stopped, but Dianne was still having contractions. She was exhausted. Decision: to call the doctor. We drove to the clinic and the doctor examined her. There was still no change. He suggested that we wait an hour.

It was three o'clock in the morning. I saw no point in waiting any longer and decided that we should go immediately to the hospital. The doctor concurred, and we left for the hospital just as the snowstorm hit. We didn't talk much on the way. Everyone was exhausted except for me, and I had to pay close attention to my driving. We had planned for John to drive, but when it came down to it, I felt safer in my own hands.

Once we arrived at the hospital, the doctor took over direction of operations and I discovered suddenly that I was too tired to stand. I tried to stay awake, but once Dianne was installed in the labor room and all the testing machines were connected, I had to sleep. Our doctor called in the surgeon, and sometime in the early morning, after trying pitocin, he decided they would have to operate. Fortunately, because Allison was a nurse, she was allowed to go into the operating room with Dianne, which I knew would be a help.

I was with Dianne as they began the preparation work, and I began to feel butterflies in my stomach. Someone suggested I have breakfast. Terrible hospital breakfast. I took a walk to the edge of town, looked at the mountains, listened to the cows moo in the frozen morning air, watched the mist rise above the river. I felt so open, so empty, so in touch with everything. I thought of life and death, of togetherness and aloneness. I walked back and went to the waiting room. Rahima was there. I was scared. I cried. I didn't know what was happening and I felt so locked away from my lover, so helpless.

Then suddenly, it seemed too soon, the nurse came in. I think my heart must have stopped at that second. I felt suspended in time. It seemed like a week elapsed before she said, "You have a baby boy," or something to that effect. I think I must have become immobile, because she had to ask me if I wanted to see him.

I just can't think of how to describe what happened to me when I first saw him. I had my baby and my wife. At that point the fact that we had him in a hospital or by c-section didn't matter a hoot. With all our thinking and talking about it for months—no, actually for years—there was no way that I could have conceived the absolute joy I felt at that moment.

The nurse led me around to a little room off the nursery, had me wash and put a white gown over my clothes and brought Magnus to me. I told the nurse to turn the lights off and leave the room. There in the semidarkness, I pulled the covers away and touched him for the first time. I cried with joy. I laughed.

CHAPTER NINE

Spiritual and Psychological Aspects of Pregnancy and Birth

INTENTIONAL PREGNANCY

The confirmation of pregnancy can be accompanied by a wide range of emotion from elation to disbelief to depression.

Many couples become pregnant with full intention. Wanting a child and having examined their situation, they choose to stop using birth control, and each month they eagerly wait to see whether they are pregnant. They may even undertake conscious conception, trying to approach lovemaking in clarity and prayer, bringing the rituals and practices meaningful for them to the act of love and creation. There is no formula for conscious conception; awareness in the moment is all. If you are already pregnant, share what conceiving meant for you (see Seth's and Faith's birth accounts); if not, know that conscious conception can exist and explore what it might mean when the time arrives.

Other couples have to adjust to the shock of discovering an accidental pregnancy, feeling concern about their ability to care for a child, its impact on their social and financial lives, the changes in their careers, and the kind of world the child will be entering.

Wherever on this spectrum you began, assuming that by now you have accepted the reality of your pregnancy, it is important to focus as much clarity and love on this growing being as you can. *Intentional pregnancy is possible even without intentional conception.* It's a matter of taking responsibility for the process of creation in which you are involved. The time of pregnancy is an important time for bonding with your child. Bring your husband into this process, too. It's easy for him to feel left out during pregnancy, so encourage him to become involved with the baby, too, and make a point of showing him how much you love him.

CARING FOR YOURSELF AND YOUR BABY

One of the ways you can show your love for your baby is to take special care of yourself and your body; after all, it is your baby's home. Explore and celebrate your body. Take up swimming, exercise or dance, improve your diet, give up drugs, smoking and alcohol, if you use them. Treat yourself to massages. Spend time outdoors if the weather is good. Explore the resources in your community and find other pregnant women to share with emotionally and through activities (doing massage, swimming at your local recreation center, etc.)

Pregnancy is a time of tremendous emotional openness, a time of transition, growth and maturing. Although at times having your emotions so close to the surface may be distressing, it also means they are more accessible to you. You can undergo change if you are willing to feel them, without indulging yourself, and allow them to be transformed. *Pregnant Feelings* has been written as a self-help guide for exploring your own inner landscape.

SEXUALITY AND BODY IMAGE

Some women's interest in sex increases markedly once they are pregnant and no longer feel a subconscious resistance each time they make love. Other women, however, find that most of their sexual energy seems to be going into making a baby.

Whatever changes go on in your body and your psyche, communicating with your partner is the key to a loving, caring relationship. If you, like many women, find it hard to communicate about what goes on in bed, you might open discussion by both reading *Making Love During Pregnancy*, by Elizabeth Bing and Libby Colman, a beautifully illustrated book in which couples talk about their changing sexuality.

There are no medical restrictions on making love during normal pregnancy. As long as the waters haven't broken, you can't hurt the baby. The important thing is that both partners are comfortable and enjoying it. (The one exception is that if you have a history of miscarriages you should probably desist during the times when you would have had your first few periods). As your belly gets larger, you will of necessity have to explore other positions for intercourse. It's also a good time to explore other things that are pleasurable to each other, whether other ways of having orgasm or of enjoying pleasuring each other without concern for climax. Hormonal changes and increased incidence of vaginal infections may make intercourse uncomfortable for you, but it doesn't mean that you have to stop being intimate in other ways. As always, try to communicate about what you are both feeling before it leads to resentment and crises, and try to give to each other as much as possible.

GETTING CLOSE TO THE BIRTH

As your due date approaches, you may suddenly find that the baby, and the fact that you're about to be a mother, become real to you. All of the preparation we have discussed should help you feel better able to meet the challenges of giving birth. But you still may find that doubts and questions remain, so talk them out with your partner, your birth attendant, or with a friend who is a good listener. If you have questions or feelings that don't resolve with more knowledge, trust your intuitions.

Before you give birth, I recommend that you resolve all past births, abortions and miscarriages. Any unresolved emotions from past experiences can inhibit or otherwise influence your labor and birth experience. Use whatever method you know for handling psychological issues: contemplation, meditation, analysis, reliving the events, etc. If you have no method, try writing down what happened in detail, then burn the pages as you say "good-bye" to any pain or suffering in those experiences.

There are many things that can help you be ready for the birth, but "right attitude" is perhaps your best preparation. Feel and maintain your conviction that birth is a normal physiological process to which your mind and body are well-suited. This basic faith in the normalcy of birth, combined with your own level of responsibility in preparing for it and commitment to be with each event as it unfolds, should lead to a joyous, fulfilling birth experience. A little stage fright is common and healthy, for you are facing an unknown experience, one that involves a fundamental life process and that will leave no part of you untouched.

ESPECIALLY FOR FATHERS (BY WAHHAB)

Becoming a father is a major change of state, much as becoming a husband is. Unfortunately, our culture provides almost no preparation, support or even recognition of this change. (Even paternity leave, which scarcely confronts the real issues, is still more a hope than a reality.)

The key to the process is the willingness to be more mature and more responsible, both closer and less demanding in your loving, more giving and less self-centered. In short, becoming a father is an invitation to growth if you are prepared to accept it. If you are not, then discord, disagreement and suffering result.

An unfortunate view of modern popular psychology is that relationships are supposed to be fulfilling. Not only is this institutionalism of self-centeredness contributing to the breakup of many families, but also it is in direct opposition to a spiritual approach.

I am convinced that love and service are the true keys to the human process of spiritual transformation. They originate on a higher level than the self-centeredness which dictates most human actions, and they enrich the world instead of depleting it, touching people far more deeply than other acts. Consciously conceiving, bearing and raising a child is the primordial example of love and service.

I find that applying these ideals of love and service to my own life has led me to a position which could be described as radical feminism. I cannot feel that by performing one fragment of the tasks that face us as a family (e.g., earning some money) I am therefore somehow exempted from other tasks. Love never takes a vacation! Instead, I am dedicating my life to the effort to respond to the needs of every situation in which I find myself. It is not an easy task, but immense gifts seem to come unexpectedly in return.

If you and your wife can consciously agree to open yourselves in service to being parents, and especially if you can carry this intention and the intensity of your love into the act of sexual intercourse as you undertake having a child, I feel this will allow you to transcend ego faster than thousands of mantras, asanas, or other overtly spiritual practices done in an attainment-oriented way. Even if the birth is close at hand, your conscious decision to be parents opens the doorway for your child to enter into a sacred family life.

Pregnancy is a time of opening, loosening, changing. For this reason it is an excellent time for growth for both of you. Probably your wife would much rather have you take a day off without pay than to work on Saturdays to get more money for the baby. Focus on human values, strengthen your union, commit yourself more fully. Your wife will have periods of emotionality, sentimentality, irrationality. At the same time she is speaking from a deep earth-borne wisdom, if only you will look past the surface of her words. Do not argue; you may disagree, but the sense of unity must override any petty differences.

You can help prepare for the birth by reading this book, taking birth classes with your wife, and practicing with her faithfully. Discuss your mutual feelings about the birth (who should be there, how it should go, etc.). You cannot predict what will happen, but you can enter the labor with a spirit of togetherness. Your maintaining a state of love, clarity and strength throughout the labor is one of the keys to your wife's being able to handle the tremendous energy which birth involves. Your coaching will be your wife's touchstone to confidence during the powerful intensity of her contractions. Also, because she may not be able to articulate her feelings well during active labor, you have a responsibility to maintain awareness of the entire situation. If you see that someone present is interfering with the energy, you might give them some task to do or ask them to leave, and you will be actively involved in any decision to go to the hospital, should it arise.

If your wife is like mine, she will try not to complain about her added responsibilities and the demands which the birth has made on her. She also may not be capable of lining up additional help for herself. Take responsibility for seeing that she has help every day for the first week after the birth. And I suggest that you take charge of more of the domestic tasks yourself—there's more for everybody to do now.

Most fathers I know are entering into much closer relationship with their infants than fathers traditionally have done. My only suggestion about fathering is to examine our cultural dictum that the mother is primarily responsible for the children. Since "helping out" only strengthens this division, we need to keep exploring if we are going to discover a new, more meaningful definition of what it means to be a father.

Our task as men is a difficult one. There are hundreds of recent books written for women to help them through the radical changes our culture is starting to undergo, but almost none written for men. And at a time when traditional family patterns are falling apart, it is both a challenge and a responsibility to be entering into a family relationship. Because of the pivotal nature of this time of transition, you and your family are necessarily explorers and pioneers. May you be blessed in this undertaking.

PSYCHOLOGICAL ASPECTS OF THE BIRTH EXPERIENCE

A woman births with both her mind and her body, and psychological factors often determine how labor progresses. Birth is not an isolated event, but a part of a continuum, an integral part of your psychological and sexual lives as a couple.

HUSBANDS AND WIVES IN LABOR

Birth is fundamentally a creative act, as is the act of sexual union. The quality and intensity of the energy present and the ultimate surrender during both events are closely related. LeBoyer's film *Birth Without Violence* opens with a darkened screen and the sounds of a woman . . . making love? No, about to deliver a baby. Indeed many women have described giving birth as intensely pleasurable and have discussed it in orgasmic terms, while many obstetricians, on the other hand, have never even noticed that there is a change in the energy level during a birth.

Our recent foremothers probably would not have described birth in sexual terms, but then pregnant women did not go out in public due to the sexual connotations of pregnancy, and men were traditionally excluded from the birthing room, just as sexual intercourse took place in the dark. With our changing attitudes toward our bodies, nudity, modesty and sexuality, it is not surprising to find more and more women enjoying labor and birth with their husbands just as they have enjoyed the sexual experience. It's hard to have birth *not* be part of the continuum of your lives, unless you put yourself in a sterile environment which tries to block out emotional, sexual and spiritual qualities. If you don't much like your body and keep your underpants on during labor, you probably aren't going to have a labor which you would describe in sexual terms (and it may be quite long, as well). On the other hand, if you and your partner feel good about sharing energy together, hugging, kissing, and having him stimulate your nipples, your labor will not only probably go faster (oxytocin really helps!) but you'll probably have a great time (see the account of Phoebe Rose's birth following).

Making love, orgasm and giving birth are all interconnected. All relate to your attitude towards spirit and body and your willingness to feel sensation. Oxytocin is released into your system during sexual stimulation and orgasm, during birth, and during breastfeeding, which is like making love with your baby.

As discussed under "Energy and Attitude" on p. 81, a man and woman in labor form a single energy unit. Perhaps the best way to be open channels for that Life Force which is going to birth your baby is to be in harmony with one another and to give to each other. The way to have more energy is to give more.

If you and your partner are having hassles in your relationship, you should discuss them and try to have them handled before labor. Use pregnancy as a time to practice giving to each other and strengthening your union.

THE IMPORTANCE OF ENERGY AT A BIRTH

Your birth environment consists only secondarily of your physical space (which hopefully is clean, warm and friendly); more important is the love and awareness of the people present. Everyone there should have an understanding of birth and the intention of contributing something, if only attention. Being with a woman in labor is like being with a holy person—if you don't have something tangible to do to be of service, you are still obligated to maintain awareness. Having people about who are not actively participating can slow down a labor. On the other hand, people need to be able to eat and relax (or even sleep, if the labor is long). Having another room prepared for attendants and friends is a good idea.

Anyone who is anxious, who feels that birth belongs in the hospital, or who is in any way upsetting the mother should be asked to leave. If it is someone you especially wish to be there, put the person to work timing every contraction or making bread, or going for supplies; sometimes having something to do can focus energy and calm their anxiety.

The husband or coach needs to avoid getting so involved with the labor that he loses awareness of the surroundings and the energy of the people involved. He should try to feel if anything is upsetting the mother, and see that it is taken care of. Also, he may want to be alone with the mother for a while and shouldn't feel reluctant to ask everyone to go out for an hour or two.

WHO SHOULD BE PRESENT AT THE BIRTH?

Given the importance of the energy which people bring to a birth, consider carefully who you want to be present. Just as you form an essence-relationship with anyone with whom you make love, there is also an essence-relationship formed between the baby and everyone present at a birth—the more so if they are open to recognizing it.

If you want to invite your parents or in-laws, consider that generally our mothers had very different birth experiences and have different expectations about birth than we do. Make sure they are informed and comfortable with your feelings and intention.

If you have other children, you need to consider carefully whether or not you want them present during birth, or only immediately afterwards. Would you feel uninhibited with them there, able to grunt or moan? Would they contribute, or require energy? The high energy level can be upsetting to a young child, and coming in afterwards still allows bonding with the baby. If children are going to attend, they need to be prepared, and to have someone present who is there only for them.

Older children can be given explanations (with plenty of drawings and pictures) of how the baby will come out, what it will look like, and what the placenta will be like. They can be included in breathing and relaxation practices. Again, it helps to have a friend to be with them to answer their questions and tune in to their needs. They can be a definite asset, helping you in many ways.

Sometimes, however, a child may not want to be present or may go out to play just as the baby is coming. Or if it is in the middle of the night, they may not wake up. It's best not to put demands on them. Being there right after the birth will be soon enough.

As your due date approaches, you may find more and more people asking if they can be present at your birth. Everyone wants to participate in the miracle of birth, but don't feel that you have to include anyone to avoid hurting their feelings. You may want your birth to be just the two of you and your attendants. Conversely, it can be really wonderful to have a lot of friends at your birth, as I did at Faith's birth. Not only is it a wonderful gift to offer them, but also they can really help you, both on the tangible level and by offering a community of support. It's a good idea to get everyone together at your house in advance (including your birth attendants) so they can all meet one another and learn what is needed and what is important to you.

Sometimes it's a good idea to tell people you do invite that you may change your mind on the day of the birth. This gives you the freedom to see who you are, how you feel, and how your labor is going.

PSYCHOLOGICAL DYSTOCIA

This is any slowing or stopping of labor for psychological reasons. Some possible causes include:

- Your own or others' expectations that you "perform"
- Trying to control your labor
- Resisting sensation
- Someone in the environment making you feel uneasy
- Feeling restrained because of photos
- Tensions between you and your husband
- Feeling negated by an insensitive birth attendant
- Unresolved fears
- Inhibition or modesty

Deal with a long labor that feels awkward or uncomfortable by trying to change the energy. Perhaps the mother has some underlying fears that need to come out. Or perhaps someone else can see what is really happening and suggest a course of action.

In particular, if labor seems suddenly to stop, (or not

get started, the "beached whale" syndrome), try sending everyone away and ignoring the labor. Go out for a walk or get some sleep. When the mother is in active labor you can call people back.

FOCUSING ON THE BABY DURING PREGNANCY

The life of the baby during pregnancy is only just now coming to our awareness. Even inside the uterus, your baby is extremely responsive. Your baby's heartbeat and brain waves change in response to loud noises or classical music as well as in response to your emotions.[1] If you have adrenaline pumping through your system, your baby will too, willy-nilly.

Thus being in a calm, beautiful environment and maintaining emotional tranquility communicates to the baby. LeBoyer advised me to sing to my baby when I was pregnant. Your baby probably responds to subtle qualities of attention and love, and certainly responds to, and may even form an attachment to, your voice.

Take time each day to focus on the baby as a being and as a body developing inside your own. And massage your belly, especially as the baby becomes larger and more cramped. Babies seem to love to be moved around. Pressing on your belly may cause your baby to start to move, almost as if it has been awakened. Indeed, babies inside the uterus show cycles of activity with brainwave patterns resembling a less developed form of the sleep, wakefulness and dream-like states of consciousness which they show after birth.[2]

FOCUSING ON THE BABY DURING LABOR

During the labor, don't place so much attention on the mother that the baby is forgotten for long periods of time. The baby is the sole purpose of labor; indeed, it is the baby who initiates labor through an interaction of the fetal adrenals and the mother's hormones and uterus. The birth of the baby—being able to see, hold and welcome him—is not only the outcome of labor, but also its cause.

The mother can keep her focus on the baby by talking to him, welcoming him, telling him that she loves him. Others in the room can maintain a meditative space into which the baby can be born, free from projection about what he or the birth will be like, but definitely focusing on the baby and allowing for what is.

---

[1]Mortimer Rosen, "The Secret Brain: Learning Before Birth," *Harper's*, April 1978, p. 47.

[2]*Ibid.*

FOCUSING ON THE BABY AT BIRTH

To understand what the baby's experience is at birth, you can imagine, and feel within your own cellular memory, what it is like being a baby in the uterine environment. For one thing it is very secure and contained—the uterine and abdominal muscles define the baby's world for it and the contractions throughout labor gently massage it. The amniotic fluid provides a warm, aquatic environment in which the baby floats suspended by the umbilical cord like an astronaut in space. In its dark, warm home the baby is constantly in motion, rocked by the mother's movements and breathing even when she is at rest. And the lullaby of the mother's heartbeat is always present, as well as other internal body noises and muffled sounds from the outside world.

Dr. Frederick LeBoyer's recognition that the newborn's cry is one of anguish and suffering led to his realization that making the baby's change of environment as gradual as possible can prevent most of the psychic trauma associated with birth. Everyone has by now probably heard of the "LeBoyer bath," but rather than espousing any set techniques, what LeBoyer is saying to all of us is to focus, to feel, to be aware of the newborn as a totally sensitive new person. Everything is new for the baby. He has not yet developed the filtering and screening mechanisms that allow us to numb ourselves to noise, pollution, and the feelings of the people around us.

OUR MEETING WITH DR. FREDERICK LEBOYER: MAY 29, 1973, PARIS, FRANCE

The story of how we happened to meet Dr. LeBoyer is included in my account of Seth's birth in Chapter 2. Since he has probably contributed more than any other person to our recognition of the baby's experience in the birth process, I feel it appropriate to include here a more detailed account of our meeting.

We went to visit Dr. LeBoyer in his apartment in Montmartre. He received us very warmly and openly—a beautiful, loving man with tremendous heart. Like the baby at the end of his book, you have to smile in his presence.

He spoke English in a gentle, lyrical voice, with traces of an Indian accent. We asked him about it, and he replied that he had learned most of his Engligh in India, working with Indian and Tibetan masters. He showed us pictures of the daughter of his hatha yoga master in India; she was nine months pregnant and still able to do all of the yoga postures. (See his latest book *Inner Beauty, Inner Light.*) He emphasized the importance of exercise and of breath. He said that it was important during pregnancy to do some form of spiritualized exercise such as yoga or tai chi to open the body and the breathing. He said it is important to give the baby as much space and breath as possible while it is in the womb, and that I should be completely relaxed in front, like a miller carrying a sack. He recommended walking, singing, and listening to beautiful music while pregnant, as well as surrounding myself with beautiful objects, thoughts and sounds. He stressed the importance of consciously taking in only good impressions. He said I should talk and sing to my baby while it was still in the womb, welcoming it before it was born.

He showed us the pictures from the book he was working on *(Birth Without Violence)* and said that the English version would probably be called "Why Should He Cry?" "Ordinary birth is as painful for the child as it used to be for the mother," he said. "Must it be so?"

His answer was a firm "No," and he went on to explain that over the past seven years he had been delivering babies in a way which was painless for the baby and in which the baby did not cry as it was born. He had stopped doing deliveries in order to work on the book and the film, which we would be able to see in its next-to-final form the following day. He knew that he had to make his perceptions available to others, but he had no idea that his work would become a worldwide phenomenon, influencing millions of people's perception of birth and having such far-reaching effects on the way babies are born.

He explained that the key to a gentle delivery is realizing that babies are so much more sensitive than we are. Everything is new for them, magnified, filled with wonder and amazement. They should not be subjected to the harsh textures, bright lights and often brutal procedures of standard hospital routines. He states, "The child will tell you what to do; he is the teacher, the Lama." It was my understanding that Dr. LeBoyer was not advocating a technique which could be spelled out in steps 1 through 5. Rather, he was telling us to be totally sensitive to what the child is experiencing and let our own awareness guide us. As he described the way in which he worked with the environment and with the baby to make the delivery as gentle as possible, I felt that quality of recognition or remembrance one sometimes feels: "Of course. I know that. That's obvious." And yet I could not have expressed it before he said it, and it certainly wasn't the way in which babies were being born in any hospitals that I knew about.

He described how he helped babies to be born without suffering by lessening the onslaught to their senses. Coming into the world forces so much that is unknown onto the child that its first experience outside the womb is one of torture. Thus he conducts the birth in dim light once the head starts to crown, and in an environment of silence and calm. The baby shouldn't be jolted or hung upside down, he stated, because it is a terrible shock to the nervous system and the spine, which has been compressed and rounded for so long. In regard to the baby's starting to breathe, he said that nature works well without us; the breathing will start, despite the anxiety we project onto the child. He said we need to listen for the breath, to allow the breathing to come naturally. And then, once the baby is breathing, to tell him that everything is all right, and that I am all right, and to radiate calm.

He then showed us the pictures of the baby being immediately placed on the mother's belly, because of the importance of skin-to-skin contact. The mother touches it, reassuring it, and the doctor or father gently massages the baby. I asked him about the type of massage, and he replied that everything is governed by the child and is in response to its needs. He said that he was doing precise things when he touched the baby's back, but he didn't go into them. I suspected that he was working with the subtle energies along the spine, but didn't pursue it any further.

I asked about cutting the cord, and he replied that once it had stopped throbbing (not before five or six minutes), it could be cut. The immediate cutting which is so common in most hospitals forces the baby into lung breathing much more suddenly than if the placental circulation is allowed to continue. It's much more a crisis and shock to the baby than if the transformation to breathing air occurs gradually, as nature intended.

He then showed us the pictures of the baby being gently held in a bath of skin-temperature water. The baby is once again weightless and free in the water. Perhaps about ten minutes old, this baby begins to explore, to move, to laugh. Seeing the pictures and experiencing babies in this bath is quite amazing. The experience in the bath, like the picture of the day-old baby at the end of the book, must cause us to reexamine and redefine our concept of the "normal" newborn. It seems that we must constantly reevaluate our concept of what the human species is capable of being.

Then, he continued, after the baby is finished in the bath, after he or she has fully opened and released (perhaps five minutes), the child is left completely by himself for a few moments. He is near you, but is allowed to feel that he is himself, a separate person. "Realize," he said, "that you are his mother, his servant, but he is not your child." Then the baby is put to the breast and allowed to nurse.

I asked him about the use of ritual and ceremonies at the birth. One of the things I was especially interested in was the developing of new rituals and celebrations which have meaning today in marking the important events of our lives. At first he said that he didn't want to give an opinion, but then he said that rituals were there to remind parents what a momentous event each occurrence is for the child. As an example, he said that eating solid food is nothing for us—we have become blasé through repetition. But the child, when it eats solid food, has an entirely new experience. So there is a ceremony, such as the one in India when the child first eats rice, to remind the parents of the newness of the moment. "We are trapped by our memory, which thinks that everything is the same," he said. "The child has little memory, so each moment is new."

We saw his film the next day. It showed me so clearly that babies were meant to be born serenely. We returned to London the following day, and unexpectedly found ourselves back in Los Angeles a few weeks later. We kept in correspondence with LeBoyer about progress on his book, its translation into English, its publication, and the progress of my pregnancy. Here are two of his letters.

TWO LETTERS FROM DR. LEBOYER

(October 1, 1973)

My dear,

Last point: you are expecting a baby yourself. Maybe my publisher will be able to give me a copy of the book soon. And then I can let you have one so that it helps you through your own delivery. Can you read French? And do you need any "refreshing course" or do you have a clear memory of what you saw on the movie? If you want a few lines, just let me know.

In a way it is all very simple: keep clearly in mind that what is making birth a terrible experience for the baby is that all kinds of new sensations are experienced "all at a time, each one with extraordinary power." Therefore it is all very simple to avoid the "trauma of birth." Let the baby enter this world as slowly as possible, that is to say let him go from one new experience, that is, type of new sensation, to the next and make these new sensations as mild and progressive as possible.

Inner sensations: Breathing. Therefore do not have the cord cut as soon as the baby is out. Keep the cord intact as long as it keeps beating. Why? You will have all that in the book.

Outer sensations: I° Silence: do not talk and ask all people around to keep silent. If you have some training in meditation there ought to be no difficulty. And then you cannot but know that words are not necessary for communication or rather for communion. Do not talk with your mouth but talk with your heart.

II° No light. As soon as the head of baby is out switch out the lights and keep only a candle or so.

III° Touch. No one can imagine the sensitiveness of a newborn. There is only one thing the skin of the baby can tolerate for the first moments and that is skin. Your skin. Therefore have the baby put on your lap. No napkin or anything of the kind. It is a skin to skin it wants. Then put both your hands on the baby very lightly in order to make him feel: "I am here. I am here. Mother is here. Mother is all right." Yes: Mother is all right. For the newborn has the feeling that in the struggle of being born mother has been killed. For, indeed once baby is out and nothing holds him tight any more, there is an unbearable feeling of aloneness and being utterly lost.

Once cord stops beating, the next thing the skin of the baby will tolerate is water. Have a small bathtub full of warm water (temperature of the body) prepared and have the baby immersed. The back of the head of the baby is to rest on the wrist of the obstetrician or the nurse. Baby is merely to be supported in water like anybody learning how to swim or rather to float.

Keep baby in water as long as all tensions in his body have been released. There ought to be no tension at all and baby ought to play, stretch arms and legs with an evident pleasure. Then only have baby taken out of water, dried and wrapped up in warm things and left to himself for at least five minutes. Certainly you want to have him and pet him. That is you want to enjoy. Let "him" enjoy. Let the baby enjoy being on his own and experience for the first time in his long life (there is already a long, long past of nine terrible months), let him enjoy that for the first time nothing is moving any more. The tempest is over and all is still and quiet.

My dear if you keep all this clear and let your doctor know, your child will be blessed.

All the very best.

F. LeBoyer
1-10-73

Seth Kenner Baldwin was born at home in Los Angeles on November 1, 1973. He weighed 8½ pounds, breathed immediately, and was the first baby born in America using LeBoyer's insights. He never cried, and really relaxed in the bath which Wahhab gave him. Dr. LeBoyer wrote back on November 21:

Thank you for the nice card and the good news.

Do you know that this boy of yours was born on the same day as I was born myself! Therefore he cannot but. . .

For the time being you cannot but be terribly busy with this baby and you cannot but give him all your time. So we shall not talk about the book or the film or lectures for the time being. Let us keep that in mind for later on. But I am so glad it was of some value and help to you.

I am going to Iran on Sunday. It so happens that there is an International Film Festival there, that the Queen has seen the film and has invited me to go and present the film and introduce this new approach of childbirth!

I shall be back in Paris by the beginning of December and anyway, as soon as the book comes out you will have a copy.

Once again all the best for both of you and the happy little one.

F. LeBoyer

FOLLOW-UP STUDIES OF THE BABIES LEBOYER DELIVERED

We asked him how long he had been doing birth this way, and what the long-term effects on the children were. He said that at that time he had been doing it for seven years, and that the children carried with them a certain calmness and strong sense of self and weren't afraid of the dark or timid in other ways.

Since then, the French Journal *Psychologie* has published results from the first follow-up study on "LeBoyer babies" completed in 1976 by Daniel Rapoport. They provide the first clinical verification of the hypothesis that birth is our primary formative experience which affects the rest of our lives.

Rapoport tested 120 babies in groups of forty, consisting of one-, two- and three-year olds, which were chosen at random from among the thousand babies delivered by Dr. LeBoyer in a conventional Parisian hospital. Sixty percent of the women in the study were working mothers, mainly office or factory workers, skilled craftswomen or employed in small businesses. None was personally acquainted with Dr. LeBoyer or his methods before her baby was delivered. Sixty-five percent had never met him, while 35 percent had become aware of his methods during their prenatal visits. Thus for the majority, it was only with the onset of labor that they received an explanation of the silence, lowered lights, and other procedures that he was going to use. The results were as follows.

All the infants scored substantially higher than the average baby on the Brunet and Lezine test for psychomotor functioning. In general, they walked earlier than the average infant, at 13 rather than 14 or 15 months. No significant difference was detected in their language ability.

The mothers described their children as extremely alert, adroit, inventive, and ambidextrous. The fact that a "LeBoyer baby" is commonly ambidextrous suggests specifically that our split-brain functioning, with the left lobe usually predominant, can be traced to the severe feeling damage which the average newborn needlessly suffers.

Of the 120 mothers, 112 reported a complete lack of problems in toilet training and in the child's learning to feed itself. And 107 of the babies had no digestive or sleeping disorders of any kind. Various doctors who are favorable or opposed to the technique have reached the same conclusion: "Children born in a serene and peaceful way seem to be secure, in their first months, from such psychosomatic symptoms as colic, as well as the paroxysmic crying associated with a neonate."

It is only possible to use LeBoyer's suggestions if they feel right in the moment, not for any imagined gains in the future. LeBoyer has been faulted for having the obstetrician do the bath, but it is easy enough to have the father do it at the mother's side. His view that the baby experiences labor as a terrifying struggle with the monster mother was no doubt his own memory as re-experienced in analysis, but such feelings are certainly not universal.

FOR FURTHER READING

Birth Without Violence, by Dr. Frederick LeBoyer. Remembering and experiencing what birth is like for the newborn, with suggestions for making the transition as gentle as possible. An artistic book.

The Experience of Childbirth by Sheila Kitzinger. One of the first childbirth educators to deal with the psychosexual aspects of pregnancy and birth.

Making Love During Pregnancy by Elizabeth Bing and Libby Colman. Couples telling about their changing sexuality. Helps you realize you're not alone.

Pregnancy as Healing by Gayle Peterson. A holistic approach to growth during pregnancy.

Pregnancy: The Psychological Experience, by Arthur and Libby Colman. Based on the authors' pregnancies, research, and experiences of bringing pregnant women together in support groups.

Pregnant Feelings by Rahima Baldwin and Terra Palmarini. A companion volume to this book designed to explore the psychological aspects of pregnancy and giving birth.

Spiritual Midwifery, by Ina May Gaskin. One of the earliest books focusing on the psychological and sexual aspects of labor and birth.

Transformation Through Birth by Claudia Panuthos. An excellent book on the emotional and growth aspects of pregnancy and birth.

You Are Your Childs First Teacher, by Rahima Baldwin. The nature of the incarnating child and parenting experience from birth through age six.

THE BIRTH OF PHOEBE ROSE

Mary Ann Montoya

Prelude:

We had our first baby, Jacinta, at home two and a half years ago. My contractions were so intense that I did fast transition breathing the whole eighteen hours. I was very skeptical that any other breathing would help on this second birth, but was inspired by Rahima's classes and reading *Spiritual Midwifery* (Gaskin) to try a slow breathing technique. I got the ideas for the birth mantra (the power of saying "I love you") and hugging and kissing to help open me up from the same book. I am now convinced that love and tantric touch are the keys to easier birth.

Story:

Victor and I woke up around 2 A.M. and couldn't go back to sleep, there was so much energy in the room. I figured it was just a strange case of double insomnia, when suddenly at 3:25 I had an amazing contraction that felt suspiciously like the Real Thing. Contractions continued every five minutes and I assured Victor that this was our baby's birthday and we should call the people we had invited to our birthing (my doctor had told me I was already 4 cm dilated on my last exam).

Victor and I were really excited and began to kiss and hug a lot, especially during contractions, and we told each other lots of "I love you's" to open me up.

Pretty soon I decided I'd better think of a method to help relieve tension because Victor was my "midhusband" and had lots of things to prepare for the birth. I remembered reading in the *Informed Homebirth Newsletter* of gripping two combs to activate reflex points in the fingertips and palms for an easier birth. So I positioned the combs for the next contraction and was amazed at how they relieved the discomfort and at the same time seemed to open me up.

We continued to love each other a lot and I felt we were helping the baby to be born into an atmosphere of love, in addition to helping me relax. Victor looked just beautiful to me and I felt him lend me all his energy to help me birth this baby.

I started losing my sense of time and space as my rushes were getting much stronger. I decided, instead of any set breathing pattern, to begin saying a mantra of exactly what I wanted to accomplish in each rush. One I used the most was "I'm opening up real wide. . ." I would concentrate deeply on the meaning of the words and believed the power of the spoken word would do just that. Concentrating on the words centered my attention and seemed to regulate my breathing perfectly.

It was important to me that I relate each rush to my baby's birth as a whole and not feel each as an isolated entity as I had experienced with my first birth. Saying the mantra really seemed to accumulate and build energy throughout labor and mushroom that energy for the beautiful, intense experience of birth itself.

Whenever I felt I needed extra control for a contraction, I found saying, "I love you" to Victor or God or the baby or the friends in the room really focused my attention and opened me up even more.

I loved being in the bathtub and spent transition there. My contractions were overlapping each other, and Rahima and Victor were right there, encouraging me, being quiet with me and giving me energy. I still had my combs clutched in my hands and said mantras through every rush. I also found gently and slowly rolling my head to the rhythm of my rushes and mantras kept my shoulders and neck relaxed.

Jacinta, our two-year-old, woke up and was happy we were having our baby today. LaVerne took care of her and fed her and helped her to feel relaxed about all the high energy that was buzzing in the house.

My last few rushes of transition were intense, and I found it helpful to simply say, "I'm going to relax." It felt good to say something as basic as that, as I was getting very spaced out.

Suddenly I felt the energy begin to change, and I knew it was time to get out of the tub. After a while of lying on the bed, I got up to urinate once more and had a huge rush which broke my waters.

I got back on the bed and Victor massaged my perineum with olive oil to help stretch and relax me. I waited to have a strong urge to push again and since I didn't, I decided to try squatting on the bed. With the next contraction Phoebe came down and almost crowned. Rahima reminded me to lie down and pant-breathe to prevent tearing. I waited as I felt Phoebe push against my perineum and finally I reached down and pulled myself gently apart and her beautiful head was born.

She was born breathing, but pretty blue-looking compared to Jacey's birth. The cord was loosely around her neck and slipped over her head with the next contraction. On that next rush daddy Victor caught her beautiful 8¼-pound body.

He laid her on my bare belly and she fussed quietly. I held her snugly with my hands to reassure her. She quieted. We all loved each other and her.

Jacinta loved Phoebe right away and climbed up on

the bed to touch her and kiss her. We all watched in amazement as Phoebe Rose changed into rainbow colors, so rosy and perfect and wonderful.

Victor cut the cord, and I squatted for the placenta. Phoebe was nursing well which helped my uterus to contract. Everyone had breakfast, which tasted *so* good.

Postlude:

I was completely astounded by the birth. I was amazed at the effectiveness of the power of the words "I love you" in generating love among us and the power of saying exactly what I wanted to accomplish in each rush. And clutching the combs really helped me relax. I had a five-hour labor compared to a marathon eighteen hours with Jacinta. The quality of the entire birth expe-

rience was extremely high, with much more concise and focused energy using these methods.

We all still feel the magic of our birth and the magic of life in our little Phoebe.

Love was made more perfect in all of us because of Phoebe.

Mary Ann Montoya

Note: Second babies are *easier, but I was astounded by this birth, too. The input from* Spiritual Midwifery *really helped Mary Ann's labor, and I felt privileged to have shared with them in such a high experience. It also felt really good to all of us that Victor and Mary Ann stayed in charge and delivered the baby themselves.*

Rahima

CHAPTER TEN

The Newborn

THE NORMAL NEWBORN

You've been in relationship with your baby for many months of pregnancy, communicating with him on an intuitive level, but what will your newborn look like? Many parents are expecting their baby to look like the ones in baby-food ads. However, these babies are usually three months old—your newborn will look quite different!

The first view you will have of your baby is usually the top of its head. As it starts to appear at the vaginal opening, you may wonder how anything so wrinkled, gnarled and bluish-grey can relate to a baby. The *molding* (overlapping of the skull bones) as the baby passes down the birth canal causes the gnarled appearance, and the head may be elongated or otherwise oddly shaped when the baby is born, but the molding usually starts to go away within the first few hours and will probably be nearly gone by the end of the first day.

As the baby slips out, you may be amazed by his bluish color and the slippery, shimmery energy surrounding him. As you watch, the baby will take his first breaths, marvelously turning pink, starting from the chest area and extending to the extremities. Your baby's thermal regulatory system is still immature and it's important to keep him warm (e.g., next to your skin and covered with a receiving blanket that can even be warmed in the oven if it's winter time). Your baby doesn't need to cry at birth in order to make the change from placental circulation to lung breathing. The process can occur gently in the first few minutes after birth, but the baby does need to "pink up" well. The change-over in the circulation, closing of the heart valves, etc., requires many hours or even a day to be completed.

You will probably notice that your baby's head is quite large in relation to the rest of his body, and his arms and legs are small by comparison. The average newborn weighs about seven pounds and is about twenty inches long. His nose is usually quite flat and his ears may be flattened against the sides of his head from passage down the birth canal. But he really *is* beautiful—and not just because he's your baby! Babies have a certain purity that can remind us of our own essential nature.

Many parents know in advance whether their baby will be a boy or a girl, and they seem to be as often right as completely surprised. Your baby's genitals may be quite enlarged at birth; this may also be true of the breast tissue, in boys as well as in girls. Both these factors are due to the high levels of hormones in the mother. Girl babies may even have a bit of vaginal bleeding during the first month due to the mother's hormones, but it soon stabilizes.

Your baby may be born with only a small amount of *vernix*, or it may be covered with this cream-cheese-like substance, which keeps the baby from turning into a prune in the amniotic fluid. It is very good for the skin, and can be rubbed in rather than washed off. The amount of vernix seems to relate to individual differences, although postmature babies tend to have less. Areas of the skin may also be covered with *lanugo* or downy hair which usually falls out in the first week (more common in premature babies).

The newborn's skin is usually pink or reddish in color, and it is normal for it to peel in the first few days after birth. Even babies whose parents are black, oriental or American Indian have light skin; the pigmentation spreads from a bluish area on the lower back, and the baby will darken as it gets older.

Newborns often have *milia*, or small white spots on their faces. These are caused by oily material retained in the pores before the sweat glands open up. They will go away within a week or so and should be left alone. Babies may also have "stork bites" on the back of the neck, eyelids or forehead which are caused by the rupturing of small groups of capillaries during birth. There are sometimes small hemorrhages in the whites of the eyes, too; they are harmless and will start to clear up within a few days. Dark purple birthmarks on the skin will not go away, but are also harmless.

IS MY BABY ALL RIGHT?

Within five minutes after birth, your baby should be doing very well according to the five signs which Virginia Apgar developed for evaluating the newborn (see p. 69 for the Apgar scoring). The five areas are as follows.

Breathing. Babies breathe rapidly during the first few hours after birth (60–70/minute), and then the rate slows to about 40–60 breaths per minute. Breathing should be fairly regular and not require an undue amount of effort. If the baby remains mucousy, suction him out and lay him on his side for the first few hours so mucous can drain naturally. Giving the baby a few drops of sterile water to drink can also help to loosen mucus.

Color. The baby should be completely pink, including the hands and feet, lips and ears.

Muscle Tone. The arms and legs should show good flexion and movement.

Reflex Response. The baby should be responsive to touch. For example, touching the cheek should produce the rooting reflex, and suctioning the baby should produce a grimace.

Heart Rate. The newborn's heart rate should be between 120 and 160 beats per minute. If it is not, and especially if it is below 100, notify your doctor.

Your baby should continue to breathe well and have a good strong cry. It should have good eye-to-eye contact and nurse well.

EXAMINATION OF THE NEWBORN

The important consideration is that your baby is healthy, and that any problems are spotted as soon as possible, either by you or your doctor. If you are going to be seeing a pediatrician regularly, find out if he will come to the house, or plan to take your baby to be examined within the first day or two after the birth.

You will want to check over the baby yourself shortly after birth. It's not necessary to do an entire medical examination, just focus on the baby, letting your attention go from head to foot. Have the room warm, take the baby's diaper off, and use your eyes and your ability to observe the obvious. Use your intuition. If something is bothering you, get it checked out, either to find out what is wrong or to put your mind at rest.

Before beginning, be familiar with the section on the normal newborn so you know about molding, skin color, etc. Then look for the following.

DANGER SIGNS IN THE NEWBORN

If your baby has any of these signs, refer to the explanations following, and check with your doctor or take the baby to the hospital if necessary.

- Failure to breathe well:
  Blue skin color (including extremities, lips or nails
  White skin color (body is pale and limp)
  Grunting with each exhalation
  Retraction of the chest
  Very rapid breathing (more than 70/minute)
  Flaring nostrils, very difficult breathing
  Gasping for breath
- Meconium in the water
- Jaundice in the first 24 hours or very yellow at 3–7 days
- Lethargic baby, failing to nurse; lack of reflex responses

- Heartbeat below 100/minute
- Convulsions
- Profuse, excessive salivation
- Distended abdomen or bladder (not urinating within 24 hours or not passing meconium within 48 hours)
- Vomit that is bile-stained
- Bloody stool (not to be confused with a spot of vaginal blood in girl babies)
- Any obvious birth defects:
  Openings along the spine or back of scalp
  Extremely low ears (associated with kidney defect)
  Cord not having two arteries and a vein
  Cleft palate or lip: check before baby nurses
  Dislocation of the hip; club foot
- Fontanelle bulging or deeply sunken when baby at rest

MECONIUM IN THE WATERS

If the waters broke and were stained with meconium, but the heartbeat was strong and you delivered at home, the baby should be thoroughly suctioned as soon as the head is out to prevent meconium aspiration syndrome (meconium being inhaled into the lungs, resulting in pneumonia or death). Watch for respiratory problems. Have the baby checked by a pediatrician.

SKIN COLOR AND BREATHING

If your baby has not pinked up by the five-minute Apgar scoring, you should be taking emergency measures. If the baby is pale and limp, keep it warm, suction it immediately and apply CPR. This can be done on the way to the hospital if necessary.

If your baby is breathing but his extremities or the area around his mouth remain blue, you should see a doctor. Again, keep the baby warm.

Respiratory Distress Syndrome (RDS) is a serious complication. Signs of it will usually occur within a few hours after birth, but they may come on within a day or two; they are most common in premature infants.
- Rapid breathing (more than 70 breaths/minute a few hours after birth)
- Labored breathing; flaring nostrils when inhaling
- Grunting when exhaling
- Gasping for breath
- Retraction of the chest (the chest goes in under the ribcage or between the ribs when breathing)
- Continued blueness of the skin, extremities, lips or nails

GENERAL WELL-BEING OF THE BABY

Your baby should continue to breathe well and have a good strong cry. It should have good eye-to-eye contact and nurse well.

LOW BIRTH WEIGHT

If your baby weighs less than five pounds, it may be either premature or small for gestational age (SGA) and should be checked by a physician. Because of the complications which plague premature infants, the baby should be checked for signs of prematurity (perhaps you missed a period before becoming pregnant and the baby is younger than you had thought). Common complications involve hyaline membrane disease of the lungs, hypoglycemia, and acidosis in the blood. If the baby is term (37 weeks or more, which can be verified through physical characteristics and reflex responses), then you will probably be able to care for him at home, although SGA babies can also have blood sugar or developmental problems.

One couple in my class had a second baby under five pounds (their first had been only a few ounces larger). The pediatrician they saw said that, even though it was term, if they didn't put it in the hospital within an hour (where it could be in an incubator for two weeks) he would report them for child abuse. They were really upset, then exercised their legal right to ask for a second opinion and found a pediatrician who thoroughly checked the baby and let them care for it at home, bringing it back daily the first few days to check certain areas of concern. This doctor even made a house call. Their baby was fine and wasn't subjected to the isolation of an incubator. Because your baby seems so small and helpless, it's hard to remember that you still don't have to give up your responsibility and decision-making abilities to outside authority.

THE HEAD

1. We have already discussed the molding common to newborns. Many babies, especially firstborns in which labor has been long or difficult, are born with a slight swelling called a *caput succedaneum* (Figure 10-1). It consists of serum which has accumulated, and it crosses the suture lines of the skull (where the bones of the head join together). It should start to go away immediately after the birth and is usually gone within 24 to 36 hours.

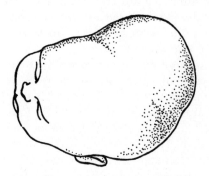

FIGURE 10-1. *Caput succedaneum.*

If the swelling appears within the first few hours after birth and does not cross the suture lines of the skull, it is probably a *cephalohematoma*, which contains blood rather than serum, and takes weeks or months to disappear. Neither is very serious, but you can have them checked out if they are very pronounced.

2. The *fontanelles* are the two soft spots where the skull bones join together. The back one is often not too noticeable, but the front one stays soft up to eighteen months of age, by which time it should be closed or a

doctor consulted. When the baby is at rest, the fontanelle should neither sink way in (a sign of possible dehydration) nor bulge upward (a sign of possible internal pressure within the cranium). If the front fontanelle is nearly closed and the suture lines are quite calcified, the head may not be able to expand for the growing brain, so check with your doctor.

3. Defects along the midline of the scalp or along the spinal column are called dermal sinuses; they are vulnerable to possible infection or meningitis. More serious *closure problems* along the spinal column include spina bifida, in which hair covers or surrounds the hole, or myelomeningoceles, in which the nerve tissues protrude from the hole. Do not touch them. Apply a piece of sterile gauze, and get the baby to the hospital.

4. A *Down Syndrome baby* (one suffering from the chromosomal anomaly once known as Mongolism) is more common in women over forty and is usually recognizable from physical characteristics: the eyes have a fold giving them an Oriental appearance, the upper lip is short and the tongue is thick and fissured, and the fingers are stubby with clear-cut "simian lines" on the palms. Mental retardation is almost always present, and the baby should be seen by a doctor.

5. A baby may have congenital kidney immaturity if it has very low-set ears, a broad nose, and receding chin.

6. A cleft lip is obvious and can usually be corrected surgically. A cleft palate can be noted by looking or feeling inside the baby's mouth. If the baby's tongue is protruding, it can be an indication of brain injury. If the baby salivates profusely, it may have tracheoesophageal fistula, in which the alimentary canal dead-ends and there is an opening into the windpipe, or cystic fibrosis. See your doctor!

7. Discharge from the eyes on the first, second or third days would probably be the result of chemical burning if silver nitrate had been used in the eyes.

Discharge on days 2 to 5 might be indicative of a gonorrheal infection if silver nitrate or antibiotic had not been used. Take the baby in and have the discharge cultured immediately if you have not used eye drops at birth; antibiotic treatment through injection can be effective if the infection is caught early.

Other types of eye infections are common during the first two weeks. If you have any doubts, have the discharge cultured so it can be diagnosed and treated.

THE NECK

Check the neck for masses and hematomas.

THE CHEST

The chest should be evenly shaped. Again, check the breathing—it should be between 40 and 60 breaths per minute. Check the chest sounds with a stethoscope. Breathing should sound about the same on the top and bottom of each lung. Check the heart rate—it should be between 120 and 160.

THE ABDOMEN

The bladder shouldn't be distended, and you shouldn't feel any masses in the abdomen.

GENITAL AREA

The genitals may be swollen; girl babies may have a spot of blood from the vagina. See if the boy's testicles have descended. The baby should urinate within 24 hours. The urethra should be visible. The anus should also be visible and the baby should pass meconium within 48 hours.

JOINTS AND EXTREMITIES

1. Check all the fingers and toes. The legs and feet may curve in slightly due to the position in the uterus, but you should be able to straighten the feet out.

2. Check for dislocation of the hip (incidence: 1 in 1000, six times more common in girl babies). With the baby on her back, bend the knees and grasp the thighs with your thumbs on the inside (Figure 10-2). Rotate the thighs so that the knees come together and spread apart, usually touching the table. If movement feels unequal, or if you hear a click, there may be dislocation and the baby should be seen by a doctor. It can usually be corrected if found early. Also turn the baby over and check that the folds of the legs are symmetrical and that the legs are both the same length.

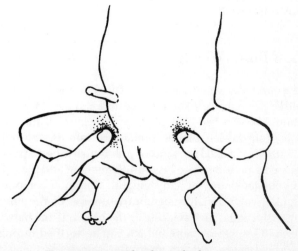

FIGURE 10-2. *Checking the hip joints.*

OVERALL ASSESSMENT

Check your feelings and reaction to the baby. Does the baby seem to be healthy? Is there something that is bothering you? Who can give you further information?

WHAT TO EXPECT
FROM YOUR NEWBORN

Your baby will communicate with you through its various kinds of cries, through eye contact, and through some kind of intuitive faculty. This wordless link is so strong that you'll find yourself waking up at the same instant as the baby, and there really isn't any danger of rolling over on the baby if he sleeps with you. Tune into what the baby needs—he may be hungry, wet, tired or just bored. Hold him, rock him, talk or sing with him, and once he can sit up you can carry him around in one of the soft baby packs that keeps him close to you, lets him view the world as he gets older, and leaves you with both hands free.

When your baby is alert and active, just enjoy being with him. You don't have to *do* anything special, just be in relationship with this new being, and don't forget the importance of touch. Ashley Montague's book *Touching* reminds you to baby your baby while he *is* a baby, so he will be able to grow into maturity as he gets older. You can't spoil a baby, and you really can't touch them too much. (I also recommend Joseph Pearce's book *Magical Child* which gives a spiritual/scientific view of a child's development.) One of the advantages of the infant seats so popular now is that the baby is allowed to *see* what is going on rather than being stuck away in a crib or playpen, but a disadvantage is that they don't allow him to *feel*. Using a baby carrier or a shawl as they do in Latin America enables your baby to be incorporated into your life and to be in direct contact with you.

Even at birth babies can focus on and track a bright, contrasting object if it moves slowly. They can make eye contact with you, and this is especially important during the first few hours of life. Investigate the laws concerning the use of silver nitrate in your state; it may be you can use something like Ilotycin which doesn't burn the eyes as much but still prevents blindness in case the mother has gonorrhea. Whatever you use, you might want to wait a few hours before putting the drops in the eyes, so the baby can focus clearly without chemical burning.

Your baby is sensitive to sound and can turn towards it. Sudden loud noises or the feeling that he is about to fall will cause the baby's arms and legs to fly up in a startle reaction, and the baby may also start to cry. This is called the Moro, or startle, reflex. Babies don't need absolute quiet, however, and if you get your child used to living and sleeping with normal noises of your household you won't have to turn your life inside out because of the baby. Babies do need to be kept warm while they are tiny, but they don't require that you go tiptoeing around them. Your baby is also very sensitive to light, so it is good to keep extremely bright lights away from him.

In fact, all of your baby's senses remain highly attuned so care should be taken throughout early childhood. Everything a young child experiences is taken directly into its body, and is related to later health or disease of various organ systems. Be aware of where you take your baby and what impressions reach her.

During the first or second day your baby will pass meconium, the thick, tarry substance which is in the newborn's intestines. After that, if you are breastfeeding, your baby's stool will probably be mustard-colored and quite loose; it has little or no odor (unlike bottlefed babies). Your baby should also urinate during the first 24 hours, although it often does so during the birth process and this may be missed in the flurry of activity.

Hunger and digestion are earth-shaking events for the newborn. The entire world becomes these hunger pangs or the bubble of air as the baby's digestive system tries to cope with all the new processes. One of the great advantages of breastfeeding is that the baby doesn't have to wait while a bottle is being prepared. Feeding on demand, rather than according to someone's idea of a schedule, means that the baby's needs are immediately satisfied—a firm foundation for the setbacks of later life! Your baby may want to nurse continually, or he may only nurse for five minutes on each side until the milk establishes itself.

Your baby will sleep quite often, and you should use the opportunity to rest, too. However, many babies today sleep much less than books describe our generation as having done, perhaps because of the drugs and trauma we went through at birth. Our definitions of normal keep changing as our ability to be in tune with ourselves and our children increases. For example, babies aren't supposed to be able to smile until they are about two months old, yet many of our babies are smiling at one and two days old (see the picture at the end of LeBoyer's *Birth Without Violence*). Or consider the Ugandan babies who are born at home and never leave their mothers' sides. These babies have head-neck control and eye focus at 48 hours, crawl at six to seven *weeks*, etc. Ugandan babies born in a Western hospital in that country follow the same development pattern as European and American babies, so it is not a racial difference that is involved.[1]

---

[1] This and other fascinating studies can be found in Joseph Pearce's *Magical Child* (NY: E. P. Dutton, 1977), p. 38 ff.

Each baby is unique, and the more you can tune in to your baby's rhythms, the easier it will be for the two of you to be together. Comparing your baby's development with a friend's baby or with your own older children does not allow him to be a unique individual.

RELATING WITH YOUR BABY

Your baby will probably be alert and responsive for a little while after the birth. He can and does show remarkable interest in the outside world. The hours and days immediately following the birth are an important time in forming the relationship between parent and child. It's the time to fall in love with your baby, and this process of bonding occurs not only between mother and baby, but also between the father and the baby, and with brothers and sisters as well.

Some hospitals are even establishing "bonding rooms" in which families are allowed to be together, a difficulty that doesn't need to be overcome in a home-birth! The current focus on bonding is primarily the result of studies by Marshall Klaus and John Kennell.[2] One of their studies showed that when mothers were allowed an hour of skin-to-skin contact immediately after birth, and over the next three days spent fifteen more hours with their baby than the regular hospital group, significant differences became apparent. At one month the early-contact mothers showed:

- Greater soothing behavior
- More eye-to-eye contact and stroking during feeding
- Greater reluctance to leave the baby with someone else
- Greater attentiveness

Mothers who had early contact with their babies had fewer problems with breastfeeding, held their babies more confidently, and even a year later tended to touch and cuddle their babies more in a stress situation than did the control mothers. At two years, differences were noticeable in the ways in which the two groups of mothers spoke to their children: the early-contact mothers used more adjectives and twice as many questions while the control mothers used twice as many commands.[3]

At home you don't have to worry about being allowed to be with your baby. Just be with her, recognizing her as a separate person, and realizing that babies relate very strongly through touch and smell.

Although they are also able to focus and make eye contact, you convey your love and your emotions primarily through your touch: the way you hold her, the way in which you change her diaper, and through breastfeeding. And breastfeeding also releases hormones in your body, which stimulate your maternal feelings toward your baby.

Fathers who are involved with the birth process also form a close bond with the baby, and many fathers have held their baby skin-to-skin right after the birth, or taken the baby into the bathtub with them.

BREASTFEEDING

Pediatricians and even formula companies have been forced to agree that "breast is best." Certainly the advantages of breastfeeding are enormous, and there is no reason why any woman can't breastfeed with good information and support. Contact La Leche League at 1-800-LA LECHE and read the books mentioned at the end of this chapter to get a good start.

Breastfeeding provides your baby with milk ideally suited for her growth and development, as well as being

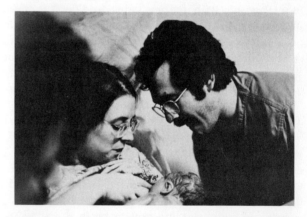

FIGURE 10-3. *Letting the baby nurse right after birth.*

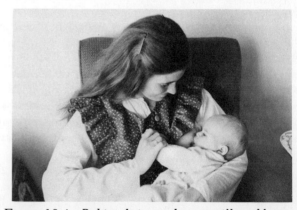

FIGURE 10-4. *Babies thrive on breast milk and love.*

---

[2]Marshall Klaus and John Kennell, *Parent-Infant Bonding* (C. V. Mosley Co., 1982).

[3]Quoted in "First Concerns in the Postpartum Period," *Patient Care*, February 1, 1975, p. 68.

a way of touching and loving your baby. Your skin, your smell, your touch, the taste of your milk and the reassurance of sucking and feeling you close to her (even hearing your heartbeat again and hearing your familiar voice) provide a continuum of security for your baby, from which she will gradually grow to explore the rest of the world.

Breastfeeding starting right after the birth is also good for you, because it releases oxytocin which causes your uterus to contract and go back into shape. And it assures your frequent, loving contact with your baby.

BEFORE YOUR MILK COMES IN

The first and most important step for successful breastfeeding is latching your baby onto the breast correctly. *The Womanly Art of Breastfeeding* details the technique in chapter 4.

Correct positioning—with your baby's belly tight across yours and most of your areola (not just the nipple) in his or her mouth—can go a long way toward preventing sore nipples. Nurse frequently, on both sides each time.

The first milk your baby receives is a creamy yellow substance called colostrum. It is high in protein, helps flush out meconium and prevent jaundice, and contains leukacytes to give your baby immunity to many illnesses.

WHEN YOUR MILK COMES IN

The more your baby sucks, the sooner your milk will come in. La Leche League and the American Academy of Pediatrics state that breast milk is all your baby needs for 4 to 6 months. It is normal for mammalian babies to lose weight during the first few days, and to regain their birth weight by about seven days after birth. If your baby seems dehydrated, however, you can give him some sterilized water with a spoon.

By the third day your milk will probably come in. Because nature doesn't know you didn't have twins and wants to assure your baby's survival, your breasts may be overfull (engorged) and be very tender. Nurse your baby, remove some of the pressure by expressing some of the milk with your fingers. Take the entire areola between your thumb and first finger, moving your thumb toward the nipple and squeezing the milk out. Move your hand all the way around the nipple so that you drain all of the ducts which lead into the nipple. Or you can buy a simple breast pump at any pharmacy.

Your baby will probably want to nurse every two hours at first. Breast milk is very easily digested since it is your baby's natural food. Your baby will probably never follow the four-hour schedule of bottle-fed babies. If allowed to nurse on demand, your baby will gradually find his or her own rhythm. And the convenience of being able to tuck the baby in bed with you for the night feedings is wonderful!

COMMON MYTHS OF BREASTFEEDING

What If I Don't Have Enough Milk?

It's unlikely you won't have enough milk if you are feeding your baby on demand and giving no supplements or pacifiers. The size of your breasts has no relationship to your ability to nurse your baby (although there may be a relationship to how much they leak in between feedings). The amount of milk you have is dependent on how much the baby sucks. If your baby is dissatisfied, let him feed more often and suck for longer each time and within 48 hours you'll have more milk. Giving him a bottle will mean that he sucks less, which will actually cause you to have *less* milk (and because it is easier to get liquids out of a commercial bottle, your baby may become lazy and not want to suck so much at the breast—don't give any bottles or pacifiers during the first month unless you absolutely have to).

Another way you can make sure your milk supply is good is by drinking plenty of fluids, eating well, and resting. Brewer's yeast is especially good for increasing your milk supply.

What If My Milk Isn't Rich Enough?

Your milk is ideally suited for nourishing your baby. If it appears thin and watery, it is because the milk rich in fat content doesn't come down until later in the feeding.

What If I'm "Too Nervous"?

The way in which the milk gets to your baby is through the let-down reflex. When your baby sucks, oxytocin is released in your blood system, which causes the milk sacs in your breast to contract and squeeze the milk into the ducts so your baby can get it out. The tingling sensation you may feel in your breast at the beginning of nursing, or sometimes between feedings, is this reflex at work. It is involuntary, and you may experience it when you hear your baby cry or even think about him (milk may even leak from your breasts then).

Tension or worry can inhibit this reflex, so see what might be happening in your environment. Perhaps someone is making you uncomfortable or undermining your confidence; perhaps you're not getting enough rest. Sit back, with lots of pillows, drink some milk or juice, and relax. Your baby and your body know what to do.

might be happening in your environment. Perhaps someone is making you uncomfortable or undermining your confidence; perhaps you're not getting enough rest. Sit back, with lots of pillows, drink some milk or juice, and relax. Your baby and your body know what to do.

SOME PROBLEMS OF BREASTFEEDING

Flat or Inverted Nipples

If during pregnancy your nipples appear flat or are inverted, spend about five minutes a day grasping the nipples between your fingers and trying to get them erect by rolling them around. Your partner can also help by sucking on them. I also recommend wearing breast shells (not nipple shields) a few hours each day during pregnancy.

Sore Nipples

If, despite your best efforts to position your baby correctly, you still find yourself with sore nipples, you can speed the healing process by nursing in a variety of positions and keeping your nipples dry.

Let the nipple be exposed to the air by sitting outside in the sun, or by at least keeping the flaps down on your maternity bra. Avoid drying soaps or alcohol; avoid plastic-coated pads in your bras. Let the baby nurse for only ten minutes at a time on the side that is sore.

If you are attentive to sore nipples, they will probably not become cracked. A cracked and bleeding nipple may mean that you need to stop nursing from that side for a few days, exposing it to sun and air and hand-expressing

milk from it. If you are having difficulties with breast feeding, contact your local La Leche League leader for advice and moral support.

Sore Breast

This is your body telling you to slow down; rest is essential. Go to bed with your baby, if at all possible, and apply hot compresses to the nipple, soaking loose secretions which may be plugging the duct. Let your baby nurse often and longer on that side. Keep the breast empty and the milk flowing through it. Plugged milk ducts are soon relieved with plenty of rest, heat, and frequent nursing.

Breast Infection

If soreness or a tender spot, lump, or red streak on your breast remains, and you have a fever or flu-like symptoms (feeling tired, nauseous, run-down, or achy), you may have a breast infection. See your doctor, finish *all* medication if prescribed, continue to apply heat and get plenty of rest. Nurse often; the antibodies in your breast milk will protect your baby from bacteria and the infection will disappear more quickly the emptier the breast. Contact La Leche League for further information on avoiding a repeat infection.

TAKING CARE OF YOUR BABY

YOUR BABY'S SKIN

Getting a good start with breastfeeding will go a long way toward helping you feel confident in your ability to take care of your baby. The main things your baby needs are milk, warmth and love.

You don't need to wash the baby as soon as it's born. The vernix is very good for the skin and can be rubbed in. You will want to wash off any blood from the baby's head and from the folds under the arms, in the creases of the legs, etc.

Your baby's skin may peel shortly after birth, and she may develop a sucking blister on her upper lip. The adjustment from an aquatic to a terrestrial life is a big one!

Babies are quite prone to rashes during the first few weeks. You might want to make sure you are using non-allergenic laundry soap, and it sometimes helps to keep a cloth diaper under the baby's face when she sleeps. The diaper is soft and can easily be changed if the baby drools or spits up, without having to change the entire crib sheet. Newborn rash *(erythema toxicum)* often appears on the face, neck or shoulders. There's not

---

CONCERNS IN THE FIRST WEEK

If you notice any of the following in the first few days after birth, check with your doctor:

- Infection around the cord (oozing, foul-smelling, redness)
- Baby lethargic, failing to nurse
- Jaundice in the first 24 hours
- Pronounced jaundice on days 3 to 7
- Blueness in the extremities or lips
- Breathing problems
- Projectile vomiting
- Fever or below normal temperature

Get answers to any question you may have or anything you feel uncomfortable about.

much you can do about it, but I found that using a little baking soda mixed with water seemed to help my children.

Another common problem which newborns often develop is cradle cap, a yellow, flakey growth on the scalp. The cure and prevention is to keep the head very clean—washing it every day and giving it a good brushing with a soft baby hair brush seems to work quite well. If the scabs get particularly thick, they can be soaked off with a bit of oil, but usually water is sufficient.

The baby's skin is so sensitive that many mothers prefer not to put paper diapers or rubber pants on their newborn. Keeping a rubberized "puddle pad" underneath the baby prevents a wet crib and allows air to reach the baby's skin. If your baby does develop diaper rash, the best cure is always sunshine and fresh air. Just leave the diaper off for a while. Lanolin or an organic oil is probably best if you need to keep the diaper on or if the irritation isn't too bad. Petroleum-based products rob minerals from the skin, and creams or ointments with too many perfumes or chemicals can increase the problem. An excellent line of natural baby-care products including herbal soaps, calendula cream, powder, etc. is available from Weleda, Inc., 841 S. Main St., Spring Valley, NY 10977.

TAKING CARE OF THE CORD

The cord should be kept dry and above the diaper. Alcohol can be put on the cord once a day to help prevent infection and to dry it. It should fall off within a week after birth.

Until the cord falls off, give the baby sponge baths rather than immersing him in water. If you do the LeBoyer bath, make sure the tub is clean and that you are confident of your water's purity.

The cord should be dry and not bleeding. If it is bleeding it can be retied with a sterile shoelace. Use alcohol on it daily to keep it disinfected. If the discharge is foul-smelling, or if the stump is wet after a day or so, there may be an infection. Redness around the stump extending in lines or redness along the abdomen is another sign of infection. See a physician, as you would for any sign of infection.

JAUNDICE

Physiological jaundice of the newborn is quite common, with between a third and half of all babies showing slight yellowing of the skin. It is only a problem if it becomes severe. Symptoms occur around the third to seventh day, when the baby appears yellowish or tan in color. When you press on the forehead with your thumb and then remove it, the blood recedes, but the yellowness caused by the jaundice will be evident.

The yellow appearance is caused by the presence of unconjugated bilirubin in the blood from the breakdown of red blood cells which the liver is unable to handle effectively (the baby in utero has more red blood cells than it will need after birth).

The extent of the jaundice is usually determined by a blood test. If the bilirubin count gets as high as 12 the situation will require close supervision and phototherapy (treatment with particular wavelengths of light). The danger is that if the amount continues to rise, the baby can experience brain damage. An exchange transfusion is usually done when the bilirubin is greater than 20 mg/100 ml on a baby less than 5 days old. If the baby is older, they may wait until the bilirubin reaches 25, treating it first with phototherapy.

If only the head seems to be affected, the bilirubin count is probably low; if the head and chest are affected, the count is probably 6–12. If more of the body is affected, the level is quite high and should be tested.

The eyes are also an indicator of the severity of the condition. If only the corners of the whites of the eyes are yellow when the lids are pulled away, the jaundice is probably quite mild. If the whites of the eyes appear yellow when looked at straight on, the condition is more serious.

If you see your baby starting to become jaundiced, the treatment is to place him in the sun or under fluorescent lights with his eyes protected. Keep him there for about 10 minutes on one side, then on the other. The light acts on the bilirubin in some unknown way, helping the body to excrete it. Also, nurse frequently. The baby may need to be roused to nurse, which can be done by using a cool washcloth on the cheek or forehead.

If the condition seems to involve more of the body, or if you don't get rapid improvement from the lights, get a blood test through your doctor, pediatrician or health department. Have another test done after twelve hours to see if the level is increasing, decreasing or stabilized. The treatment in hospital utilizes fluorescent lights and blood tests every twelve hours, so find out if you can set up the lights at home and take the baby to the lab for tests, or if you can remain with your baby and nurse him if he does need to be hospitalized. Jaundice can become serious, so it is necessary to pay attention, but it is also good not to be separated from your baby during these first two weeks. So contact a sympathetic pediatrician (through La Leche League or friends) if it looks like your baby will require treatment in the hospital.

If the jaundice occurs within the first twenty-four hours, it is not physiological jaundice and requires immediate medical attention. Causes might be Rh or ABO blood incompatibility or infection in the newborn.

Breastmilk jaundice is extremely rare and usually occurs around the fourteenth day. It is not necessary to give up breastfeeding permanently, although it may be necessary to stop for two or three days to let the bilirubin level come down. If this happens to your baby, contact a La Leche League leader, as well as a pediatrician who is supportive of and informed about breastfeeding.

PKU TEST

Almost all states require that a PKU test be done to detect babies with phenolketonuria, a rare enzyme deficiency which can result in brain damage and death, but which can be successfully treated by diet if diagnosed early in life. Blood is usually taken from the baby's heel and analyzed. The best time to do it is when the baby is between one and two weeks old. In the hospital they do it before the baby is released, but now many hospitals are recommending that it be done again after a week, since the baby needs to have digested protein in order for the test to be accurate.

Vitamin K is necessary for blood clotting, and hospitals routinely give injections of Vitamin K to prevent the rare cases of internal bleeding that might occur before the baby manufactures its own Vitamin K. One pediatrician I talked to felt that the mother's natural bacteria on the breast helped the baby's system to make this vitamin, so the risk was not very great if the mother was breastfeeding.

CIRCUMCISION (BY WAHHAB)

If you are going to circumcise your boy baby for religious reasons, then you have the dictates and rituals already defined for you. "This is my covenant, which ye shall keep, between me and you and thy seed after thee: Every man child among you shall be circumcised." (Genesis 17:10). Be present at the *bris* and participate in the experience and significance which it carries for you.

Where there are not religious reasons for circumcision, however, there has unfortunately grown up what in my opinion is a pseudomedical argument for circumcising for health. Circumcision is definitely painful and upsetting to your child. The arguments of hygiene are not well-founded if the child is taught to pull the foreskin back and wash his penis. And it is not, in my opinion, justified to make the baby go through a painful operation just to make his penis look like Dad's (unless *you* feel there is something wrong with an uncircumcised penis). Although I have read many arguments on

both sides, the decision seems usually to be based much more on emotional than on factual issues. If, however, you decide to have a circumcision, I strongly recommend that both parents participate in the process with strong awareness of their intention.

Even the American Academy of Pediatricians has finally stated that there is no medical reason to circumcize a baby, and that the foreskin should *not* be pulled back in uncircumcized babies until it works its way back naturally, usually by the time the child is four years old. Many pediatricians still force back the foreskin of a newborn, which is very painful and should not be done. You can request a copy of "Care of the Uncircumcized Penis" from the Academy of Pediatrics, Publications Dept., P.O. Box 927, Elk Grove Village, IL 60007.

The entire topic seems to be clouded by a lack of knowledge; as always, you'll have to bring as much of yourself as possible to bear on the issue and make your own decisions.

REGISTERING THE BABY

If your child is likely to attend public schools or get a passport, you will probably want to get him a birth certificate. Contact your local public-health department or county clerk after the birth. Usually they will send you the form by mail, although you may need to return it in person. Registering your birth also contributes to accurate reporting of normal homebirths, and will balance those being recorded which ended up going to the hospital.

FOR FURTHER READING

Breastfeeding by Sheila Kitzinger or *Bestfeeding* by Renfrew, et al. Best new books!

Circumcision: The Painful Dilemma by Rosemary Romberg. Extremely detailed account of all aspects of circumcision, its historical development, care of the uncircumcized child, etc.

Touching by Ashley Montagu. A very readable book on the importance of tactile experience for human survival and development.

The Well Baby Book by Mike Samuels, MD and Nancy Samuels. A holistic approach to care and development. When to get more help, and when to treat at home.

The Womanly Art of Breastfeeding by La Leche League International. Their official guide, practical and well-written.

You Are Your Child's First Teacher by Rahima Baldwin. Parenting issues from newborn through age six.

CHAPTER ELEVEN

After the Birth

HOW DO YOU FEEL?

The day after a beautiful birth a mother phoned me to ask if I thought she should go to the emergency room. When I asked how she was feeling, she said "Wonderful." She didn't have a fever or excessive bleeding. I was puzzled until I learned that the source of alarm was the doctor to whom the husband had taken the baby to be checked. Apparently he had such dire images of home-births that he was sure the poor woman must be totally ruined.

So let me repeat, "How do you feel?" You may feel very high and so energetic you can't sleep, or you may fall asleep in the middle of a sentence—either is perfectly normal. But after the birth and the delivery of the placenta you should feel *good* and all your vital signs should be normal: pulse, blood pressure, temperature; you should not feel clammy or light-headed. There shouldn't be excessive blood loss, and the placenta and membranes should be complete.

BLEEDING

The most immediate concern for your health is that you aren't bleeding too much. There will be a gush of blood when the placenta separates and more as it is delivered, but then it should pretty much stop, with the total amount of blood loss not exceeding two cups (review the section on third stage on p. 71 if necessary).

Once the placenta has separated, the open blood vessels need to be sealed off, which is accomplished by the contraction of the uterus. Once the placenta is out,

your uterus should feel hard and firm, about the size of a grapefruit, and be below your belly button. You'll feel contractions every time you nurse, and there may be a spurt of accumulated blood then. These "after contractions" can be uncomfortable with second, or subsequent, babies because your uterus has been stretched more, but they should be welcomed as nature's way of restoring your internal balance.

You should also have someone massage your uterus every ten or fifteen minutes during the first hour after the delivery of the placenta. Have them push quite deeply on the sides of the uterus and/or rub up from the pubic bone to stimulate a good contraction; don't push down on the top of the uterus, because it can strain the ligaments and result in the cervix coming out of the vagina. The uterus should feel hard and firm. Feel it yourself—it's the only time you can feel your nonpregnant uterus all by yourself. It should remain hard even after your birth attendants have gone home.

Once it is clear that the initial bleeding has been stopped, the placenta should be examined to make sure it is complete (see Chapter 5). If a piece is retained inside the uterus, there will be continued excessive bleeding as well as the danger of infection and later hemorrhage. There may be "extra pieces" passed, which are actually blood clots, and shouldn't be cause for alarm; what you are concerned about are pieces *missing* from the placenta. If you have any question about the amount of blood loss or the integrity of the placenta, take it with you to your doctor or emergency room of the hospital.

If you're soaking two sanitary pads in half an hour, you're bleeding too much and should have it checked out. You may have a slow-trickle hemorrhage, internal tears, or retained fragment of the placenta.

TEARS IN THE PERINEUM OR BIRTH CANAL

Have you torn? Sometimes a tear is visible as the head comes out; other times a tear might be internal and be suspected because of excessive bleeding.

Examining for tears is done with sterile gloves and close attention to sterile technique. Using a good light, your birth attendant will examine the external perineum, around the clitoris, the inner labia and urethra, and the pelvic floor muscles. If there are tears that require suturing to heal well, sterile gauze pads can usually be used to control the bleeding with pressure until the suturing can be done. First-degree tears often heal well without any stitches (see Figure 8-1, p. 112, for the three degrees of tearing).

If you have torn badly and your birth attendant is not able to do suturing, you should go to your doctor or clinic to be stitched within the first six hours after the birth. You shouldn't wait until the next day or the day after that because the risk of infection is too great then (you would be stitching all of the bacteria up inside of you).

> If you are Rh⁻, don't forget to take in some cord blood to determine the baby's Rh factor and see whether you need an injection of RhoGam. You must have the shot within 72 hours for it to be effective.

VAGINAL DISCHARGE AND SECONDARY POSTPARTUM HEMORRHAGE

The lochia, or postpartum flow, may persist for several weeks. Bleeding should lessen, so that during the first few days it will be mucousy and blood-stained, similar to a period, and then it should become lighter but still be mucousy.

Around the tenth day the lochia may become white or brownish-white. However, the reddish lochia may continue for up to two weeks if small pieces of the placenta are being passed or if the placental site is not healing rapidly.

If your lochia is clear and then suddenly becomes red blood again, it is a sign that you have overdone it (too much lifting, standing, or running around). Rest and don't try to do too much too soon. Secondary hemorrhage occurs most commonly between the tenth and fourteenth days. It is most often due to a retained fragment of the placenta, but sometimes nothing has been

retained. If bleeding is heavy or doesn't stop with rest, see your doctor without delay.

SIGNS OF INFECTION

If the lochia is foul-smelling, if your uterus is tender, or if you develop a fever over 100°F, you should see a doctor immediately. It is good to take your temperature at the same time each day for the first week, and be sure not to put *anything* in your vagina as long as the lochia is still flowing. Infection can be serious and lead to death if it becomes systemic; it responds well to antibiotics, so don't sit around if you have any of the above signs.

GETTING UP

If your uterus feels firm to the touch and you are feeling able, you can get up after the birth, but take it slowly and sit on the edge of the bed for a few minutes so you don't get dizzy. Have someone with you so you don't fall. Blood will have accumulated in your vagina, so don't worry about the flow as you stand up. Have sanitary pads handy. It's good to drink something before you try to get up.

HUNGRY?

Having a baby involves a tremendous amount of energy and a tremendous loss of fluid and body mass. You will probably feel thirsty, and you should drink immediately after the delivery of the placenta, before trying to get up. Drink something such as tea with honey or fruit juice to prevent collapse. After that, eat or drink anything you feel like having.

You should urinate within eight hours after delivery so your bladder doesn't become overstretched while it is still relatively insensitive from the birth. (You may have to remind yourself to urinate, and relaxing on the toilet or running water to add the power of suggestion can help prevent an overfull bladder, which then cannot be emptied voluntarily and may require catheterization).

It's not uncommon to be constipated after the birth, and drinking prune juice can help with the first bowel movement. Also helpful is elevating your feet when going to the toilet, relaxing the pelvic floor and pushing with your diaphragm.

WHAT NOW?

The birth probably wasn't exactly what you were expecting, and you may find that having a new baby isn't what you were expecting it to be, either. Give up expectation and be willing to feel what you're actually feeling.

Use the time immediately after the birth to be with your baby, your partner, and older children if you have any. Feel yourselves as a new family. And take time to rest. I can remember sitting up on the bed holding Faith immediately after her birth and then waking up in the same position, still holding her.

Many first-time parents are nervous about how to relate with a newborn, what to "do" with him or her. Actually, the most important thing is to *be* with your new baby. Just hold him and get to know one another, allowing the love which flows through all creation to flow through you and feeling the pure energy which emanates from a baby. In one study, about one-third of the women said that they first felt love for their baby a week after the birth. So don't feel guilty if you aren't feeling what you anticipated; just stay open.

ABOUT EMOTIONS

Having a baby is a tremendously involving and moving experience. The "baby blues," or postpartum depression, is not as common with homebirths as with hospital deliveries because of the active part you have taken in giving birth, the loving environment, and not being separated from your baby or your husband afterwards. But you may still find your emotions quite strong and unpredictable, for the time surrounding birth is one of immense power and energy. You may feel at one with all creation and united with all women who have ever given birth, and you may feel terribly vulnerable and uncertain. As much as possible, be open to all that you are feeling. Something within you can be touched and strengthened through this period of time.

Some things you can do to help stabilize your emotions during the first few weeks are to get sufficient rest, eat well, have adequate help so you can be with your baby, and see that you aren't left alone.

GETTING ADEQUATE HELP

In order to rest and be with your partner and your baby, you'll need someone to handle all the chores of that first day: washing the sheets and other laundry, shopping for food, cooking dinner, straightening up the house, and so forth. Having a homebirth is an all-involving experience for your husband as well, so don't expect him to handle everything right away either. And, since paternity leave is not yet common in this country, he may have to go back to work the next day. You don't want to be left alone thinking about all the things you "ought" to be doing. Have adequate help to handle the daily chores of the first week, leaving you free to recuperate and to share with your new family.

Everyone wants to help, but many people don't know what you need, or they don't want to risk disturbing you. Make a list of everything that needs to be done, so that when someone asks, or comes to visit, you can give them something to do. They'll be glad to help.

It is hard for many of us to ask for help. We feel that we ought to be able to do everything ourselves or that we don't want to bother others. *Arrange help in advance.* One possibility is to have a friend or relative stay with you after the birth. It should be someone who is going to help with the house, not someone who is going to tell you how to be with your baby, or otherwise make you or your husband nervous. Another possibility is arranging for various friends to stop by each day between 3 and 5 P.M. to do shopping, cleaning and preparing dinner. Anyone who was present at the birth should be willing to put in a day helping you afterwards.

The need for support and help during the first week or so cannot be emphasized strongly enough. Overdoing it can exhaust you and make you miserable, as well as resulting in delayed hemorrhage. So don't try to do it alone! Relax. Be with your other children, be with your new baby, and let someone else keep the house together and feed everyone. Besides, people love to help and you're providing them with an opportunity to express their love and caring.

NURTURING YOURSELF

NUTRITION AND REST

After you have your baby you should be feeling healthy and fit, but your body is still going through major changes, not only from the birth, but also from breastfeeding. And you will find that being up at night with your baby makes napping a necessity. When your newborn sleeps, take the phone off the hook, put a sign on the door, and rest yourself. Sufficient rest is vital for a good recovery and an emotionally balanced postpartum period.

You need almost as many vitamins, minerals and protein when you are breastfeeding as you did when you were pregnant, so continue to pay attention to your eating and take your vitamin supplements. You can discontinue the iron if your hematocrit is normal at your six-week checkup.

Don't try to diet right after your baby is born. Eat a high-protein, well-balanced diet to get your strength back and watch useless calories, just as you did during pregnancy. Breastfeeding burns close to 1000 calories a day, which together with sensible eating and sufficient exercise will restore your waistline over the next few months.

Fluids are especially important for nursing mothers to establish and keep up your milk supply. Every time you nurse your baby, you should drink something yourself while your body is adjusting to lactation. Sit back with your feet up, have some pillows to support your elbows and the baby's head, and enjoy this time with your baby while you drink some juice or enriched milk. It's also a good time to share a story with toddlers or other children so they don't feel like the baby is getting all your attention.

Brewer's yeast can also increase your milk supply, and many nursing mothers take it daily mixed with milk or juice. It is rich in B-complex vitamins (often called the nerve vitamins), iron, and protein, and is very good postpartum.

Care of the Perineum

Your perineum may be tender and swollen because of the stretching it has been through, and if you have used hot compresses, you may find the area especially swollen. Applying ice during the first 24 hours can help. Place the ice chips in a "baggie" or rubber glove, cover with a washcloth, and keep inside your sanitary napkin right after the birth.

If you have torn, urinating will cause a strong burning sensation which you can lessen by pouring water over the area as you urinate. Having some betadine, well-diluted, in a bowl with cotton balls or in a squeeze bottle in your bathroom to pour over the vaginal area after urinating also helps to prevent infection and keeps the urine from burning quite so much.

Stitches can be just plain uncomfortable. They are the weakest from the tenth to seventeenth days, so don't overstretch these muscles by riding a bicycle, climbing, etc. Here are some suggestions for increased comfort.

- Lie on your stomach or your side; it may be easier than sitting.
- Take sitz baths. Make sure that the tub is clean, and let the hot water swirl around you. Don't pollute the water with soaps—take showers for cleanliness. Some sources recommend adding salt or garlic to the water to help with healing.
- Sit well back on the toilet, which can help prevent urine from stinging sore tissues.
- Hold the stitch area firmly with a clean pad when having a bowel movement.
- Homeopathic arnica or hypercal ointments can reduce bruising. Herbal compresses (such as comfrey) or aloe vera ointment can aid healing. Topical anesthetics such as Dermaplast also reduce discomfort.

Pelvic-Floor (Kegel) Exercises

You should begin doing kegel exercises (contracting the pelvic floor) as soon as the baby and placenta are delivered. It will be difficult and feel quite strange at first, but it is really important to get your muscles back into shape. Good muscle tone is vital to prevent uterine prolapse, urinary incontinence, and to contribute to sexual sensation (see Chapter 3).

Contract the pelvic floor muscles to a count of 6, hold for 4, and release. Repeat, repeat, repeat! You can also do some shorter contractions of the muscle. Do ten contractions every time you think about it: every time the phone rings, every time you change your baby's diaper, etc. You should do 200 a day for the first six weeks to get the pelvic floor muscles back into shape. Then continue kegeling the rest of your life.

What About the Rest of Your Body?

The next area of your body that will forcefully capture your attention will be your breasts, when your milk comes in on the second or third day. For more information on comfort and breastfeeding, refer to Chapter 10.

Soon after the birth it's really worthwhile to have a friend come in and give you a massage, Touch For Health, acupressure, or other treatment to help realign your body and energy flows. A chiropractic adjustment to make sure your pelvis and back are aligned can also make a big difference in how you feel.

It takes six weeks for your uterus to go back to (slightly larger than) its prepregnant size. Right after the birth you will look about the same as you did at five months of pregnancy. Your body can't adjust overnight! This entire postpartum period is a time when your body is again in transition, and any exercise you do will pay off because your muscles are wanting to go back into shape (see the program of postnatal exercise following).

If you have a checkup around six weeks, the size and position of your uterus will be noted, the cervix will be checked for any lacerations, and your blood pressure, urine and hematocrit checked. Your bleeding should be over by then, and the perineum completely healed. It's good to have the baby checked then and get answers to any questions that you may have. Know what method of birth control you want (discussed later in this chapter).

Postnatal Exercises

The following exercises are based on realigning your body and reestablishing the energy flows after labor and delivery. They also help to tone your muscles after your baby is born.

Have fun and enjoy your body as you do these exercises. It is essential that you find your own breathing pattern with your movements. Begin with just the first exercise the day after your baby is born, and each day add one or two more until you are doing the entire series. Only you know intuitively how many times to do each exercise. Be in touch with your new body. Learn to give it the same kindness and care that you give your newborn. Thanks to Sheila Sabine for sharing those exercises with us.

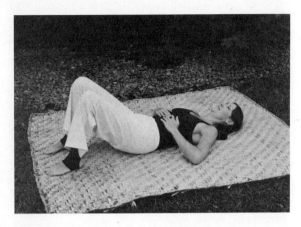

1. Lie on your back, knees bent, feet flat on the floor with palms touching rib cage. Slowly rock but do not lift pelvis. With each movement, allow small of back to make more contact with the floor.

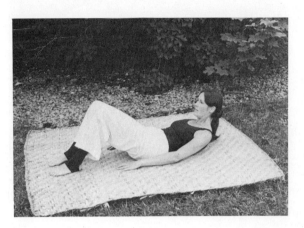

2. Lie on your back, knees bent. Contract stomach muscles and hold as you lift your head to a count of 5; then release head back to the floor to a count of 5.

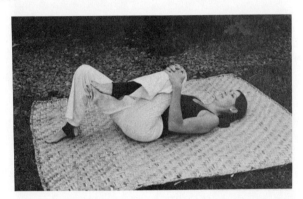

3. Lie on your back, knees bent. Draw left knee up to chest and hold for 10 counts. Release. Draw right knee up and hold for 10 counts. Release. Draw both knees up and hold for 10. Release.

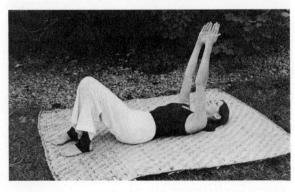

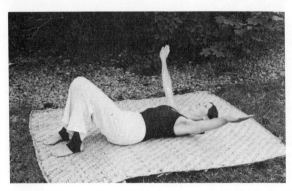

4. Lie on your back, knees bent. Slowly lift arms straight up over your head, palms facing. Turn palms outward and lower arms out to your sides, at right angles to your body, and slide palms along the floor back to your side.

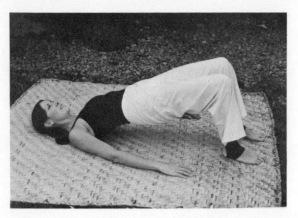

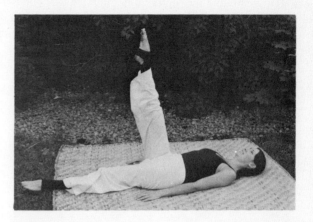

5. Lie on your back, knees bent. Slowly lift pelvis off the floor; then release, slowly allowing each vertebra to make contact with the floor.

6. Lying flat on the floor, legs straight, toes pointed, slowly lift one leg to a count of 5, release to a count of 5, and repeat with the other leg.

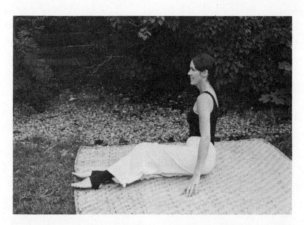

7. Sit up, legs straight out in front of you. "Walk" forward on your buttocks; then walk back.

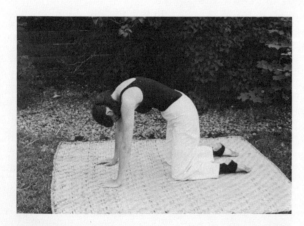

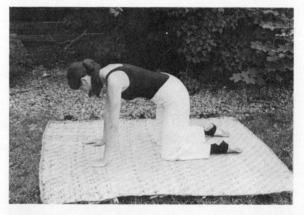

8. Get up on your hands and knees. Arms should be far enough apart so your shoulders are not tense or cramped. Arch your back upwards and pull up on your stomach muscles. Release, allowing your stomach to relax as you flatten your back.

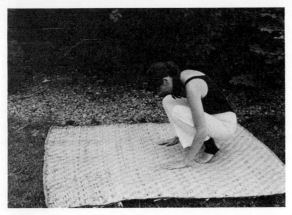

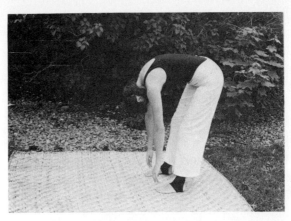

9. Get up on your hands and knees; roll back onto the balls of your feet, keeping your palms on the floor. Now slowly roll up to a standing position, keeping your head down, shoulders relaxed, feeling each body part aligning on top of the other.

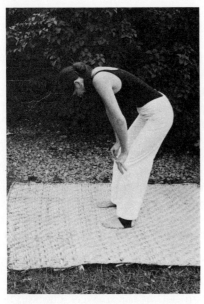

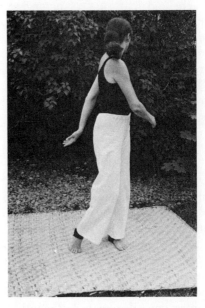

10. Standing with your feet parallel, lean over, bending your legs and placing your palms on your knees. Tighten your vaginal muscles to a count of 5, then slowly release to a count of 5. Inhale as you tighten; exhale as you release.

11. Standing with your feet parallel, arms at your sides, swing both arms to the right, rotating the upper torso and head as far to the right as possible. Allow your left heel to come off the floor as you turn. Alternate sides. Allow your body to be loose and light as you turn.

NURTURING ONE ANOTHER

Having a baby (especially a first baby, although a second baby has its own surprises) irrevocably affects your marriage. It's a big change to go from being a couple to being a family. If you are looking foward to having things the way they were, you're bound to be disappointed. Your lives together will never be the same. Surrender the way things have been, and be open to the way things are. Probably the most important thing you can do to help each other is to keep communicating about what is happening and what you both are feeling.

Since most of your energy may be going into the baby, you need to remember to give energy to your man. He may be at work all day; he may be tired and unable to handle all of the chores that have built up by the time he arrives home; he can't breastfeed the baby; and he may feel a little left out. He needs to know that he's still important to you.

And men, become involved with your baby—don't feel that caring for and nurturing children is something that's foreign to you. If you're able to be home, take on many of your wife's tasks and see that friends or relatives are coming each day to help out. It makes an enormous difference to have help that first week. Your wife may feel good, but she needs time to recover. And she really needs your care and support. For example, if you're going to be a couple of hours late coming home, call ahead, because she's emotionally very vulnerable at this time.

The weeks right after a birth are a special time, a time of closeness with each other and of falling in love with your baby and the miracle of life. But they can also be difficult weeks. Neither of you will be getting a good night's sleep, there's so much to be done, and emotions are very open and undergoing change. It is a time of adjustment and maturing, of having to accept responsibility, of always taking this new person into account and being willing to love and give continuously. It is a process of growth which we all signed up for at the time of conception—and the returns are numerous and fulfilling—but I'll be surprised if you don't feel at some point, "Nobody ever told me. . ." It's all part of the intricate pattern of life.

IS THERE SEX AFTER BIRTH?

Most women have no interest in sexual intercourse immediately after giving birth. And indeed, you shouldn't have intercourse for several weeks after the birth (doctor's used to say an arbitrary six weeks, but now the feeling is that once the lochial discharge has stopped and you are feeling like it, intercourse is fine).

Meanwhile, your husband, who probably has had less or no intercourse during the last months of pregnancy, may be eagerly awaiting the opportunity to make love again.

It's important to give to each other emotionally and physically at this time, approaching each other with tenderness and communication. Even though you may not be having intercourse, sexuality never stops; you're always in sexual relation. This is a good time to explore being sexually close without intercourse. Just as in pregnancy, exploring other ways of having orgasm or of pleasuring one another without being goal-oriented can have a beneficial effect on your sexual relationship.

When you are ready to resume intercourse, you may want to use a lubricant at first, as the vaginal area tends to be drier while hormone levels are readjusting. Some women are afraid that intercourse will hurt the first time after giving birth (tissues have been through an incredible process), but using a lubricant, lots of gentleness and communication, and actively taking the penis in and squeezing it with the pelvic floor muscles with each stroke, can make resuming sexual intercourse a pleasurable experience. Your partner should be very open to following your lead, even being willing to stop if you feel uncomfortable.

After having a baby, a woman's body image is again undergoing adjustment. She may be disappointed at how big she still is. She's wondering what her body will look like as she loses weight and her figure reemerges. Is her partner still attracted to her? What will intercourse be like? Some women have a great deal of sexual energy after the birth, while others find that breastfeeding and their hormonal balance reduce their sexual drive. Again, the important thing is to communicate with each other and to be willing to give to each other in ways that are pleasurable to you both.

BIRTH CONTROL AFTER CHILDBIRTH

Although breastfeeding without supplements for four to six months usually serves to suppress ovulation and menstruation for seven to fifteen months, it is, unfortunately, not a fully reliable method of birth control. Since you may ovulate two weeks before your first period, you will not know in advance when it occurs. First periods often occur without ovulation, but it is possible to become pregnant while breastfeeding as early as four weeks after the birth if you are not using some supplementary form of birth control. However, the La Leche League states, "Only a fraction of one percent of women are likely to conceive while wholly breastfeeding before having any periods."[1]

Birth control pills are not recommended for nursing mothers, as they affect the milk. Some sources don't recommend an IUD at the six-week checkup because the uterus is more vulnerable to perforation. A diaphragm, together with a good spermicide, is effective and has no side effects, and learning to insert it as part of lovemaking can lessen the nuisance factor. You'll have to be fitted for a new one at your six-week checkup even if you had one before, because your cervix has changed size. Or you may choose a condom together with a spermicidal foam or jelly as an interim method. Some couples are choosing elective sterilization if they have had all the children they desire, but these operations are nonreversible, so it's necessary to be sure. If you are interested in natural birth control (based on abstaining when your mucous indicates the possibility of fertility), the best discussion for nursing couples can be found in *A Cooperative Method of Natural Birth Control* by Margaret Nofziger.

---

[1] La Leche League International. *The Womanly Art of Breastfeeding* (Franklin Park, IL. LLLI, 1963), $3.50, p. 49.

BEING NEW PARENTS

THE "IDEAL PARENT"

Like most people, I had some grand ideas about being a parent before I had children: what things I would and would not do, how I would avoid all the errors of my parents and the parents I saw all around me, and how I would ensure that my children grew up according to my ideals.

But when Seth and Faith actually came into my life, the reality of the situation came as an abrupt shock. All of my idealism had in no way prepared me for the minute-by-minute, day-after-day encounter of living with a child.

Indeed, one of the myths I had inherited was that mothers should be with their children all the time, and I felt that no one could be as good a mother for Seth as I could. So that two and a half years later, when I put him in preschool because we both needed time away from one another, I felt tremendous anxiety and guilt.

And although some of the things that upset me with Seth now have a certain recognition factor when Faith goes through them in her own way, I still find that Seth is constantly forging into uncharted waters in which I sometimes sink, sometimes swim.

What is this parenting business all about, anyway? How can we turn our heartfelt ideals into daily life? How can we get beyond the roles and authoritarian models, which treat children as possessions, and still guide them? These are some of the questions which I can share with you in the unfolding process of living with children.

Our society tends to keep us isolated from young children until we suddenly find ourselves with a new baby.

Something you can do to become more involved with babies is to become friends with other pregnant couples through prenatal exercise classes, La Leche League meetings, childbirth preparation classes, or wherever. As you become friends, share your thoughts and feelings about being pregnant, giving birth, being a parent. You can help these friends by doing things for them in the week after their baby is born. And you can help a new mother, as well as learning more about being with young babies, by making yourself available for your friend to leave her baby for an hour or two while she goes shopping or does something by herself.

FREEING YOURSELF FROM OLD MODELS

Everyone wants to be a good parent and wants what is best for his or her children. Unfortunately in a time of rapidly changing ideals and realities, we tend to be the

victims of our own models. Since in fact neither we nor our children usually live up to the models of goodness which we carry in our minds, we tend to become guilty and frustrated. If you find yourself not living up to your own model, examine it as rationally as you can and see where it comes from, and if it really relates to who you are and what is being called for in your situation. It may be that throwing out your idea of what every good mother should do will put you more in touch with the real needs of your situation.

Being a parent is a complex and ever-changing process. No experts, books, or advice from others can provide you with any magical way of being a perfect parent, for our relationship with our children, like any intimate relationship, involves and expresses the whole of our lives. One key, though, that has helped me avoid unnecessary suffering when I have been able to remember it is that even though this child has come from your body and you are his or her primary care-giver from birth onward, he or she is a unique being, not an extension of you. If you take your child's successes and failures, good and bad behavior, etc., as a reflection on your character or your ability as a parent, you are setting yourself up for disappointment. As LeBoyer said to me, "You are his mother, his servant, but he is not *your* child."

ONLY THE BEGINNING . . .

Being with children is a great gift and real spiritual work if we are willing and able to rise to the challenge. They are a mirror and a constant lesson. Although most saints never had children, I'm about to institute a whole new order (with completely different qualifications) for us mothers. Having children has complicated my life about seven times over, but it has also helped me to love and to give and let me see and experience things that I never would have touched had I not become a parent. I have no words of wisdom to share with you, only my heartfelt best wishes and thanks for sharing with you in the beginning part of the adventure.

RESOURCES IN YOUR COMMUNITY

Babies and children require mothering in order to thrive. Mothers also need support if they are to be nurtured and feel good. Don't deny your own needs, and see what is available in your own community to help you in the new lifestyle you have undertaken.

La Leche League International. Monthly meetings on breastfeeding (bring your baby!). In addition to answering questions, they're a good place to make friends with women with babies, and they're a good source for information on other resources. Call 1-800-LA LECHE.

Groups for new parents. Check with childbirth educators, the Red Cross, church groups. If you don't find anything, why not organize a reunion of your childbirth preparation class, to see what can grow out of it?

Groups for single mothers. Check with the United Way, library or other community agency.

Babysitting co-ops. Especially good if they consist of nursing mothers, who can offer babies breastmilk and the same kind of care they're used to. Check with La Leche League.

FOR FURTHER READING

A Cooperative Method of Natural Birth Control by Margaret Nofziger. Detailed instruction on combining calendar, basal body temperature and cervical mucus methods.

After the Baby's Birth. . . . A Woman's Way to Wellness by Robin Lim. Mother yourself with this book!

Mothering Magazine discusses all aspects of parenting. Published quarterly—see page 52 for address.

Ourselves and Our Children by The Boston Women's Health Book Collective. Insightful book for helping us see ourselves in relation to our children.

Pregnant Feelings by Rahima Baldwin and Terra Palmarini. Contains several chapters on parenting to consider when you are pregnant and after the baby is born.

You Are Your Child's First Teacher by Rahima Baldwin. Combines the insights of Rudolf Steiner, Founder of Waldorf Education, with the practical issues of parenting the young child.

BIBLIOGRAPHY

These books have been helpful to me over the years in understanding birth and in writing this book (I have not included technical articles here, which are referenced in the footnotes of each chapter). All of these books are excellent for further reading. If you cannot find them in your area, check pages 52 and 53 for mail order sources.

HOMEBIRTH AND RELATED TOPICS

Arms, Suzanne. *Immaculate Deception*. (South Hadley, MA: Bergin & Garvey, 1985).

Cohen, Nancy Wainer and Estner, Lois J. *Silent Knife: Cesarean Prevention and Vaginal Birth after Cesarean*. (South Hadley, MA: Bergin & Garvey, 1983).

Davis, Elizabeth. *A Guide to Midwifery. Heart and Hands*. (Sante Fe, NM: John Muir Press, 1981).

Gaskin, Ina May. *Spiritual Midwifery*. (Summertown, TN: The Book Publishing Co., 1980).

Gold, E. J. and Gold, Cybele. *Joyous Childbirth*. (Berkeley, CA: And/Or Press, 1977).

Haire, Doris. *The Cultural Warping of Childbirth*. (Seattle, WA: ICEA Supplies Center, 1972).

Hathaway, Marjie and Hathaway, Jay. *Children at Birth*. (Sherman Oaks, CA: Academy Publications, 1978).

Hazell, Lester Dessez. *Commonsense Childbirth*. (New York: Berkeley, 1976).

Kitzinger, Sheila. *Birth at Home*. (New York: Penguin, 1979).

Lang, Raven. *Birth Book*. (Palo Alto, CA: Genesis Press, 1972).

Sousa, Marion. *Childbirth at Home*. (New York: Bantam Books, 1976).

Stewart, David. *The Five Standards for Safe Childbearing*. (Marble Hill, MO: NAPSAC International, 1981).

Ward, Charlotte and Ward, Fred. *The Home Birth Book*. (New York: Doubleday, 1977).

Wertz, Richard and Wertz, Dorothy. *Lying-In: A History of Childbirth in America*. (New York: Macmillan, 1977).

White, Gregory, M.D. *Emergency Childbirth*. (Franklin Park, IL: Police Training Foundation, 1958).

PREGNANCY AND BIRTH

Ashford, Janet Isaacs. *The Whole Birth Catalog*. (Trumansburg, NY: The Crossing Press, 1983).

Balaskas, Janet and Arthur. *Active Birth*. (NY: McGraw-Hill, 1983).

Baldwin, Rahima and Palmarini, Terra. *Pregnant Feelings*. (Berkeley, CA: Celestial Arts, 1986).

Bing, Elizabeth. *Six Practical Lessons for an Easier Childbirth*. (New York: Bantam, 1972).

Bing, Elizabeth and Colman, Libby. *Making Love During Pregnancy*. (New York: Bantam, 1977).

Blatt, Robin. *Prenatal Tests*. (NY: Vintage, 1988).

Bradley, Robert, M.D. *Husband-Coached Childbirth*. (New York: Harper & Row, 1974).

Colman, Arthur and Colman, Libby. *Pregnancy: The Psychological Experience*. (New York, Bantam Books, 1971).

Dick-Read, Grantly, M.D. *Childbirth Without Fear*. (New York: Harper & Row, 1959).

Karmel, Marjorie. *Thank You, Dr. Lamaze*. (Philadelphia: Lippincott, 1959).

Kitzinger, Sheila. *The Complete Book of Pregnancy and Childbirth*. (New York: Knopf, 1980).

Kitzinger, Sheila. *The Experience of Childbirth*, 5th ed. (New York: Penguin, 1982).

Kitzinger, Sheila. *Giving Birth: The Parents' Emotions in Childbirth*. (New York: Schocken, 1977).

Kitzinger, Sheila and Simkin, Penny, eds. *Episiotomy and the Second Stage of Labor*. (Seattle, WA: Pennypress, 1984).

Lamaze, Fernand, M.D. *Painless Childbirth: The Lamaze Method*. (New York: Pocket Books, 1972).

LeBoyer, Frederick, M.D. *Birth Without Violence*. (New York: Knopf, 1975).

Milinaire, Caterine. *Birth*. (New York: Crown, 1974).

Noble, Elizabeth. *Childbirth with Insight*. (Boston, MA: Houghton Mifflin, 1983).

Noble, Elizabeth. *Essential Exercises for the Childbearing Year*. (Boston, MA: Houghton Mifflin, 1976).

Odent, Michel, M.D. *Birth Reborn*. (New York: Pantheon Books, 1984).

Olkin, Sylvia Klein. *Positive Pregnancy Through Yoga*. (New York: Prentice-Hall, 1981).

Panuthos, Claudia. *Transformation Through Birth*. (South Hadley, MA: Bergin & Garvey, 1984).

Panuthos, Claudia and Romeo, Catherine. *Ended Beginnings*. (South Hadley, MA: Bergin & Garvey, 1985).

Peterson, Gayle. *Birthing Normally*. (Berkeley, CA: Mindbody Press, 1981).

Peterson, Gayle, *Pregnancy as Healing*. (Berkeley, CA: Mindbody Press, 1984).

Rothman, Barbara Katz. *Giving Birth, Alternatives in Childbirth*. (New York: Penguin Books, 1984).

Rothman, Barbara Katz. *The Tentative Pregnancy*. (NY: Viking, 1986).

Tanzer, Deborah. *Why Natural Childbirth? A Psychologist's Report on the Benefits to Mothers, Fathers and Babies*. (New York: Schocken, 1972).

BREAST-FEEDING

Gaskin, Ina May. *Babies, Breastfeeding and Bonding*. (South Hadley, MA: Bergen and Garvey, 1987).

LaLeche League, International. *The Womanly Art of Breastfeeding*. 3rd ed. (Franklin Park, IL: LaLeche League, Int'l., 1981).

Pryor, Karen. *Nursing Your Baby*. (New York: Pocket Books, 1973).

NUTRITION

Brewer, Gail and Brewer, Tom. *What Every Pregnant Woman Should Know: The Truth About Diets and Drugs in Pregnancy*. (New York: Random House, rev. 1985).

Dotzler, Louise, ed. *The Farm Vegetarian Cookbook*. (Summertown, TN: The Book Publishing Co., 1978).

Ewald, Ellen. *Recipes for a Small Planet*. (New York: Ballantine, 1973).

Goldbeck, Nikki and Goldbeck, David. *The Supermarket Handbook*. (New York: New American Library).

Lappe, Frances. *Diet for a Small Planet*. (New York: Ballantine, 1971).

Shurtleff, William & Aoyagi, Akiko. *The Book of Tofu*. Brookline, MA: Autumn Press, 1975).

Williams, Phyllis. *Nourishing Your Unborn Child*. (New York: Avon, 1974).

CHILDREN AND PARENTS

Baldwin, Rahima. *You Are Your Childs First Teacher*. (Berkeley, CA: Celestial Arts, 1989).

Berends, Polly. *Whole Child, Whole Parent*. (New York: Harper Magazine Press, 1984).

Boston Women's Health Book Collective. *Ourselves and Our Children*. (New York: Random House, 1978).

Cusick, Lois. *Waldorf Parenting Handbook*. (Spring Valley, NY: St. George Press, 1985).

DelliQuadri, Lyn and Breckenridge, Kathi. *The New Mothercare*. (Los Angeles, CA: Tarcher, 1984).

Klaus, Marshall and Kennell, John. *Parent-Infant Bonding*. (St. Louis, MO: C.V. Mosby, 1982).

LeBoyer, Frederick, M.D. *Loving Hands*. (New York: Knopf, 1976).

Montagu, Ashley, *Touching. The Significance of the Skin*. (New York: Columbia University Press, 1971).

Pearce, Joseph Chilton. *Magical Child*. (New York: E. P. Dutton, 1977).

Romberg, Rosemary. *Circumcision: The Painful Dilemma*. (South Hadley, MA: Bergin & Garvey, 1985).

Samuels, Mike, M.D. and Samuels, Nancy. *The Well Baby Book*. (New York: Summit Books, 1979).

TECHNICAL BOOKS

Apgar, Virginia and Beck, Joan. *Is My Baby All Right? A Guide to Birth Defects*. (NY: Pocket Books, 1974).

Eloesser, Galt and Eloesser, Hemingway. *Pregnancy, Childbirth and the Newborn. A Manual for Rural Midwives*. (Mexico, DF: Instituto Indigenista Interamericano, 1959).

Hallum, Jean. *Midwifery*. (New York: ARCO, 1972).

Myles, Margaret. *Textbook for Midwives*. (New York: Churchill Livingstone, 1975).

Oxorn, Harry and Foote, William. *Human Labor and Birth*. (New York: Appleton-Century-Crofts, 1975).

WOMEN'S HEALTH

Boston Women's Health Book Collective. *Our Bodies, Ourselves*. (New York: Simon & Schuster, 1973).

Carter, Mildred. *Hand Reflexology: The Key to Perfect Health*. (Los Angeles: Parker, 1975).

Deutsch, Ronald. *The Key to Feminine Response in Marriage*. (New York: Ballantine, 1968).

Nofziger, Margaret. *A Cooperative Method of Natural Birth Control*. (Summertown, TN: The Book Publishing Co., 1976).

Additional Resources

THE BIRTH DISC, by Harriette Hartigan, is a visual database of 9,000 color and black-and-white photographs illustrating the process of childbirth from pregnancy and labor through birth itself to postpartum and the newborn. The camera—accurate and immediate— documents the beauty and wonder of women giving birth and babies being born. It captures the emotions of fathers deeply caring and the joy of families celebrating new life.

To order **THE BIRTH DISC,** contact: Artemis, 3337 McComb, Ann Arbor, MI 48108: phone (313) 677-0519. Level I Videodisc: $3.00.

Also by Rahima Baldwin Dancy

Pregnant Feelings (Coauthored with Terra Palmarini Richardson). This book is unique in bringing a practical, self-help approach to the emotional and mental aspects of childbirth. Lovingly illustrated with black-and-white photographs by Harriette Hartigan. 8½ x 11, paperback, $17.95

You Are Your Child's First Teacher. A thorough discussion for parents on their special role in child development, introducing a new way of understanding both children and the human being in general, so that parents can be better equipped to be their child's teacher. Chapters include: Caring for the Newborn; Helping Your Toddler's Development; The Development of Fantasy and Creative Play; Nourishing Your Child's Imagination; Readiness for School; and more. $19.95 casebound; $12.95 paperback.

Available at bookstores or by direct order from Celestial Arts,
P.O. Box 7327, Berkeley, CA 94707 (800) 841-BOOK.

Postage & Handling: $3.50 for first book, .50¢ for each additional book. California residents add your local sales tax.
CELESTIAL ARTS, P.O. BOX 7123, BERKELEY, CA 94707

More ways to have a *Special Delivery*

- The video *Special Delivery* shows three births, one in a hospital, one at home and one in a birth center. Discussions by couples include reasons behind their choices, the role of the father, different ways of meeting fear and pain. 40 minutes VHS or BETA. $44.95

- Informed Homebirth Tape Course includes six cassettes by Rahima Baldwin covering all aspects of preparation for birth. $30

- *Special Delivery Journal,* the quarterly publication of informed Homebirth and ALACE. $20 includes a year's membership (4 issues); sample issue available for $3.50.

- Referrals to JH/ALACE childbirth preparation classes in your area. Also childbirth educator certification and birth assistant training.

Write for further information or order directly by including a check
or money order to Informed Homebirth/Informed Birth and Parenting,
Box 3675, Ann Arbor, MI 48106, (313) 662-6857.

INDEX